HYPNOSIS GUIDED MEDITATIONS AND DEEP SLEEP FOR ANXIETY AND SELF-ESTEEM

Find the Pleasure of Overcoming Insomnia and Anxiety. Take the Journey to Boost Your Self-Esteem and Calm the Mind with Hypnosis.

Copyright © 2023 by Christine Hepburn
All rights reserved.

The content contained within this book may not be reproduced, duplicated or transmitted without direct written permission from the author or the publisher. Under no circumstances will any blame or legal responsibility be held against the publisher, or author, for any damages, reparation, or monetary loss due to the information contained within this book. Either directly or indirectly.

Legal Notice:
This book is copyright protected. This book is only for personal use. You cannot amend, distribute, sell, use, quote or paraphrase any part or the content within this book, without the consent of the author or publisher.

Disclaimer Notice:
Please note the information contained within this document is for educational and entertainment purposes only. All effort has been executed to present accurate, up to date, and reliable, complete information. No warranties of any kind are declared or implied. Readers acknowledge that the author is not engaging in the rendering of legal, financial, medical or professional advice. The content within this book has been derived from various sources. Please consult a licensed professional before attempting any techniques outlined in this book.

By reading this document, the reader agrees that under no circumstance is the author responsible for any losses, direct or indirect, which are incurred as a result of the use of information contained within this document, including, but not limited to - errors, omissions or inaccuracies.

Despite the numerous benefits of hypnosis, hypnosis is not a substitute for medical attention, either physical or mental in nature. Information found in this audio-book are not intended to diagnose, treat or cure any diseases or illnesses. If you are diagnosed with a physical or mental illness or disease, consult with a qualified licensed physician or mental healthy therapist.

When listening to hypnosis recording, do so in a safe place, preferably where you will not be disturbed for the duration of your recording. You shall not listen to recordings or practice self-hypnosis while driving in a car, operating machinery, or doing anything else that requires your attention for safety reasons.

Table of Contents

Introduction *1*

Hypnosis *3*
   PRINCIPLES OF HYPNOSIS 3
   SELF-HYPNOSIS GUIDELINES 10

Introduction to Sleep *13*
   SLEEP AND THE IMPORTANCE OF SLEEP 13
   HEALTHY SLEEP – WHAT YOU NEED TO KNOW 18
   WHAT KIND OF A SLEEPER ARE YOU? 23
   EFFECTS OF SLEEP DEPRIVATION ON YOUR BODY 25
   HOW TO GET A GOOD NIGHT SLEEP 34
   HOW TO FALL ASLEEP, SLEEP, AND GET ENOUGH SLEEP 39

Hypnosis Sessions for a Healthy Sleep *44*
   GENERAL RELAXATION SESSION 44
   GENTLE GUIDED SLEEP HYPNOSIS SESSION 49
   SLEEP HYPNOSIS SESSION 1 51
   SLEEP HYPNOSIS SESSION 2 56
   FOLLOW YOUR PATH - SESSION 59
   HYPNOSIS FOR DEEP SLEEP SESSION 63

SOUNDS OF NATURE SESSION...67

COUNTDOWN TO SLEEP SCRIPT 72

HYPNOSIS FOR A MORE ENERGIZED MORNING..........................75

Meditation Explained *81*

MEDITATION AND THE MIND..81

MAIN TECHNIQUES FOR MEDITATION 85

BENEFITS OF MEDITATION, ...89

HOW MEDITATION CAN HELP YOU 89

BREATHING FOR RELAXATION..99

STRESS AND SLEEP MEDITATION..103

TECHNIQUES TO TRY OUT 106

A Path Through Meditation *112*

GUIDED MEDITATION SESSIONS 112

MEDITATION FOR BEGINNERS WITH BREATHING EXERCISES SCRIPT.......117

USING GUIDED MEDITATION FOR REDUCING ANXIETY AND STRESS 121

MEDITATION TO OVERCOME PANIC ATTACK............................125

MEDITATION TIPS FOR DAY AND NIGHT 130

MEDITATION TO BEOMING TIRED...134

GUIDED MEDITATION FOR SLEEP SCRIPT 138

GUIDED MEDITATION FOR INDUCING SLEEP 143

DEEP SLEEP MEDITATION 147

GUIDED MEDITATION THAT PREVENTS YOU FROM FEELING DRAINED AND TIRED IN THE MORNING..152

- NAPPING MEDITATION 156
- MEDITATION FOR SPIRITUAL CLEANING 160

Tips for a Deeper Sleep and a Better Lifestyle *164*
- TIPS FOR MEDITATION... 164
- RELAXING VISUALIZATION 169
- POSITIVE AFFIRMATIONS FOR BETTER SLEEP.. 172
- HOW TO FORM GOOD HABITS 179

Bedtime Stories to Relieve Anxiety and *184*

Fall Asleep *184*
- SHORT STORIES AGAINST ANXIETY AND STRESS TO HELP ADULT FALL ASLEEP 184
- FALLING ASLEEP IN A RAINFOREST-BEDTIME STORY 186
- MOTHER'S LOVE BEDTIME STORY 189
- PEACE OF MIND BEDTIME STORY... 193
- THE DREAM LIFE BEDTIME STORIES 196
- THE SECRET CABIN BEDTIME STORY... 199
- THE CUSTODIAN BEDTIME STORY 203
- JOY BEDTIME STORY 208
- BRAZIL: RIO DE JANEIRO BEDTIME STORY... 211

Conclusion *214*

Introduction

The world we live in today is a truly beautiful place to be. We may have heard many people say things like "this is a great time to be alive," and they would not be wrong. Limitless opportunities abound around us. Ranging from being able to study to having the careers we have always dreamt of and getting our dream jobs to be able to buy the things we want and travel as often as we desire, the world has so much to offer us.

Technology is also a huge part of this mix, as digital communication and social media have made it unnecessary for us to be alone. You can shop online whenever you feel like it, and you can play virtual games and immerse yourself in virtual reality at the click of a button. All these have contributed to making the world a global village that truly runs 24 hours, 7 days a week.

Due to this, we are now expected to spend every part of our days actively working to better our lives. Having some downtime is no longer considered necessary, and in some cases, you could be viewed as lazy for requesting downtime. This is both a good thing and a bad thing.

On the one hand, we are reaping the dividends of how active our society is, on the other hand, we need to consider the toll it is taking on us.

Our brains, just like computers, are not designed to be active all the time. Apart from sleeping at night (which some people do not even take seriously), there is still a lot we can benefit from taking some time to calm our minds and to relax during working hours.

Perhaps, once your head hits the pillow, all of your anxieties and worries relentlessly flash across your brain. You think about whether you locked the door, if you will meet your deadlines at work, if you are achieving the goals you set for yourself, or maybe how to achieve happiness in your daily life. These intrusive thoughts keep you awake at night and prevent your mind and body from resting. It can be agonizing to lie awake at night without the sweet relief of sleep. Furthermore, when it is time to start your day, you feel exhausted, irritable, and depressed.

If you are battling with anxiety, you actually need that downtime. You need to unplug from the continuous demands on your time and your mind and calm your mind. Doing this would change and improve the quality of your life.

At times it is easy to be so busy concentrating on yourself that you neglect to appreciate the world around you. It is easy to get caught in the trap of the mundane and the range of your own objectives, and you neglect to appreciate the excellence of life and the seemingly insignificant details.

Being progressively mindful, as well as meditating, will help you remember every single good thing with time. They would help you realize that there is no sense striving hard and feeling yourself with anxiety and then ending up not enjoying your life. Meditation and mindfulness will help you get away from the struggles of everyday life and remind you to appreciate life again by taking advantage of the beauty of the present moment.

The good part of all this is that everyone has the ability to meditate and be mindful.

Meditation and mindfulness do not need to be tedious or complicated. You can, without much of a stretch, utilize any of these methods during your day to calm your mind and keep yourself focused at the moment and free from your stressors.

Simply remember to stop on occasion and take it all in.

This book should serve as guidance to people who are having trouble sleeping and relaxing at the same time. This contains Scripts and Session to cater different problems against deep sleep. There will be many different hypnosis sessions depending on your waking times and your state of mind.

CHAPTER 1

Hypnosis

PRINCIPLES OF HYPNOSIS

Hypnosis is susceptibility of the mind to suggestions. Despite this state, a person under hypnosis subconsciously knows what is being done except that he/ she allows these things to happen.

A common application of hypnosis is hypnotherapy, which aims at improving well-being. You cannot inflict damage to a person in a hypnotized state. Even in such a state, a person can react to danger. The mind has defense mechanisms that are hard to understand.

The practice of hypnosis has been around for so many centuries. Lately, scientists devote time to study and explain how and why it is possible. Many theories arise regarding the different practices of hypnosis. Here are the truths about hypnosis.

Hypnosis Is a Natural, Inherent Trait

It happens to everyone, in some form or another. You may not recognize it or may even deny that you witness it at least once or maybe more. Every person may drift in and out of the hypnosis state.

For example, you are reading a novel. You are so engrossed with the story you do not "hear" your significant other asking you a question. Your conscious mind may not register the question, but you know you are being asked. In some way, it resembles hypnosis. Others do not call it that way.

Since it is a natural trait, a hypnotized person is not at risk of getting stuck in one state or another. They naturally drift to wake state or deep sleep. Thus, hypnosis is not dangerous. The experience is like listening to a boring speech and zoning out until the speaker finishes. Some may feel disoriented, but such feelings do not last.

Hypnosis Is Not a Sleep State

Although the word hypnosis comes from the Greek word, Hypnos, which means sleep, it does not constitute the normal sleep state. Hypnosis state seems like you are asleep, but your mind is aware, awake and responsive. You hear everything. Your senses heighten.

Hypnosis Does Not Make a Person Weak-Willed

A hypnotized person is susceptible to suggestions, but it does not mean they are weak-willed. They remain in control. In fact, they can stop hypnosis anytime they want. If hypnosis makes a person weak-willed, hypnotists could abuse such power over a hypnotized person. A lot of hypnotists could command a person to do everything they say. Fortunately, a hypnotized person remains in control despite his/her highly susceptibility to suggestions.

Relaxation Is Not a Prerequisite to Hypnosis

You can hypnotize a person anywhere, anytime, provided that person is willing. You may even do it during a strenuous activity. Hypnosis can bring relaxation, but relaxation is not a prerequisite.

Hypnosis Does Not Cause Permanent Amnesia

A hypnotist can command a person to forget, for the time being, what has transpired. This allows the mind to process the events subconsciously. In the long run, a previously hypnotized person can remember the hypnosis in great detail.

Hypnosis Is Different from a Trance State

Many hypnotists have difficulty identifying the difference between hypnotic and trance state. Most of the time, these two words are used interchangeably. The only similarities between the two are the heightened senses and highly efficient mind.

Hypnosis deals with heightened susceptibility of the mind, most likely the subconscious part. Trance state targets both the conscious and subconscious.

Hypnosis can happen to anyone. As mentioned, hypnosis is innate to all. Everyone experiences it very often. Only a small percentage of the population is not hypnotizable. Being hypnotizable is not dependent on personality traits.

Concepts of Hypnosis

Before learning the different techniques of hypnosis, you must understand the different concepts, how the mind works and how people communicate and behave. This is imperative to make hypnosis effective and efficient.

The human mind is a complex mechanism. Learning these concepts enables you to hypnotize anyone, anytime. Understanding these hypnosis concepts helps you recognize which technique to use.

Power of Suggestion

Sometimes, people act based on someone else's suggestions. This power of suggestion is what advertisers use to convince consumers to buy a product. Hypnotists also use this power of suggestion to induce hypnosis.

The most common example of the power of suggestion is the placebo effect. This is a suggestion during the waking state. Doctors, nurses, pharmacists apply this power of suggestion to patients. The doctors would sometimes give an ordinary pill to patients. Believing that this pill cures their diseases, the patients feel better. Why? The doctors suggested that the particular pill can heal them.

Combined with the power of language, the power of suggestion creates expectations. It creates a powerful way of making the hypnotized person move towards his or her dominant thoughts.

Power of Imagination

The human mind is capable of unlimited imagination. Together with the power of suggestion, you can create endless possibilities with your hypnosis.

Visualization scripts include the power of imagination. This power helps people achieve something or anything close to their physical limitations or beyond their normal capabilities.

Conscious vs. The Subconscious

In psychology, the mind can function on conscious and subconscious levels. The conscious part is what you can control. The conscious mind makes decisions, thinks logically, and performs cognitive functions. It is the origin of willpower and the recorder of short-term memory. It dwells in the past, present and the future.

On the other hand, the subconscious mind controls body functions and automatic reactions and reflexes. It does not think in executing an action. Like a computer program, once hitting the run button, the subconscious automatically executes whatever actions a particular body part or organ has to do. Examples are breathing and blinking.

The subconscious mind is the seat of habit and long-term memory. It does not change so easily. Embedded memories, actions, and reactions in the subconscious take time (or years) for newer ones to replace them. The subconscious controls self-preservation mechanisms. This is the reason hypnotists cannot make a person do something bad while hypnotized.

The mind generalizes and filters events, actions, objects or anything seen, felt, heard, tasted, and experienced. Generalization is the ability of the mind to think in blocks or concepts. It makes thinking quicker, especially in times of danger. Filtering is the ability to block sensory inputs and delete negative mental images.

Language Patterns

Hypnotists use language patterns to hypnotize other people. These patterns include dissociation, supposition, double binds, metaphors, embedded commands, exploration, and anticipation.

Use of Metaphors

Metaphorical language pattern is an excellent way to make other people trust you. They can relate to what you are saying without the feeling of intrusion to their personal lives. With metaphors, you can speak about the lives of your targets and still be confident that you can hypnotize them.

Double Binds

This language pattern offers choices, usually two, to your subjects or targets. Whatever the answer is, the outcome is the same. Most of the time the double binds language pattern is only answerable with a yes or no.

Embedded Commands

In this language pattern, you are commanding other people to do what you want them to do. It is usually used in an authoritarian method of inducing hypnosis. However, scrutinizing closely induction scripts, all induction techniques, except non-verbal method, use embedded commands to deliver suggestions and ask permissions.

Dissociation

This pattern uses an out of the body experience. Many people fall into a dissociation state when they experience stress and traumatic events. This dissociation seems to be a natural response of most people. Dissociation happens naturally during hypnosis. You can utilize this natural occurrence to hypnotize other people.

The Laws of The Mind

Thoughts affect the body. If the mind thinks you are strong, the body seems to follow. This is the reason constant emotional stress weakens the body. You can use this law to induce hypnosis. If your targets think that hypnosis is possible, they are more susceptible than those people who are skeptical.

Concentrated Attention

The more you think of something, the more it becomes a reality. For instance, constant, repeated imagination of wanting to become more sociable or efficient in work will make your conscious mind believe it. As a result, you find ways to achieve it.

However, for people who have difficulty separating between reality and imagination, concentrated attention has a negative effect. These people sometimes live in a world of protected cocoon.

In hypnosis, you can use this law of the mind to hypnotize anyone and strengthen your suggestions to your subjects. Concentrated attention makes your targets believe in anything you suggest them to do.

Dominant Effect

People create habits over time. They hold on to this habit to rationalize behavior and thoughts. Once an idea is embedded in the mind, it takes time for this to be replaced a new one. For new ideas to replace old ones, people need strong emotional connection or consequences.

Association

The opposite of dissociation, people sometimes feel when they can relate such emotions with something. For example, classical music relaxes the mind while metal rock music evokes harsh and negative vibes.

Reverse Effect

This law proposes that the conscious mind cannot force the subconscious to follow. The greater the effort of the conscious mind to understand or remember something the harder it is for the subconscious to response.

Negation

The mind does not know how to compute negation. When you say do not think of this or that, the first thing the mind does is to think of this or that. For example, do not imagine that this elephant is colored in violet. The mind interprets it as "see the elephant, it is violet."

Compounding

This law utilizes the compounding effect of repeated suggestions. Every time you make the same suggestions over and over again to the same person with only slight variations, you are creating a pattern. On the succeeding hypnosis, induction is easier than the first to third sessions.

Core Beliefs

Core beliefs are created early in life. These beliefs determine who you are and what you are in life. However, every core belief does not define all aspects of your life. One core belief may define how you deal with your social life but not how you manage your work environment.

These core beliefs are consistent with the rest of your life but can be altered through hypnosis, willpower and by other life changing events. These beliefs play a big role in retaining long term problems in your life.

Understanding these personal core beliefs will help you in knowing exactly how to hypnotize anyone.

SELF-HYPNOSIS GUIDELINES

Self-hypnosis must not be hard work. Honestly, it is much simpler than most people think and can provide almost everyone with a tool to make major changes in their lives.

There are many uses of self-hypnosis, including weight loss, smoking stoppages, self-esteem improvements, or other habits you may want to get rid of. Self-hypnosis is not just a small number of people. Virtually anyone can do it with a little training.

If we hear the word "conscious," most of us think of the brain immediately. Well, in reality, our mind has two parts, the conscious and the subconscious. About 75 percent of all our brain functions are unconscious, suggesting that our brains complete tasks without us. This goes on all day behind the scenes.

Each of us have some things, behaviors or views of life in general that we like and do not like. When we start adult life, these traits are usually unchanged because they are programmed in our early years.

The people we met, the skills we have acquired, the experiences we had all influenced our core programming. Most of us like who we are but may feel that it would be much better if we made a few changes (lose weight, quit smoking, stop biting our nails, etc.).

The biggest challenge is that although we want to change things consciously, it doesn't mean that the unconscious would encourage us. Think for a moment of a smoker. You are conscious that smoking isn't very healthy for you and will possibly shorten your life drastically. And does that mean they will because they know that leaving is clever?

No, because our sub-conscious mind still takes over (and changing our old ways is a fight) and generally the sub-conscious mind says "keep smoking" so it's smoking. The secret here is self-hypnosis. Why?

Because it gives you access to your subconscious mind and resources for re-programming it.

The first thing you learn about self-hypnosis is to simply turn your head, relax and count from 10 to 0 while you are breathing. As a result, many people will become mildly hypnotic.

You don't lose control and don't know where you are. This just means that you have reached a state of rest and relaxation in which you slow down and shut your conscious mind off. This is a step further by visualizing a peaceful place, such as a lake, forest or perhaps in your mom's lap.

The main idea here is to find a safe and secure place. By imagination, the physical, cognitive and physiological environments of our body can be affected to the same degree as if we were there. When we are in this comfortable and visualized state, our mind cannot differentiate between what is true and what isn't.

I'll not lie to you and say that self-hypnosis is really easy, and five minutes of practice makes you a master. What I will say, however, is that it is like any other skill and can be developed and perfected with good practice. You will be a guide to help you through your mind when you see a hypnotherapist.

You are the hypnotherapist with self-hypnosis and provide your own treatment. So, you choose when to start, how far to go and when to stop. It is and should be reiterated as a very important point.

Until beginning any self-hypnosis session you will decide what you want from it, how you will accomplish it and how you will feel when you're finished. It may help to write a script or construct a map of your journey. You will replay the script over and over while following the chart once in a hypnotic state. You should stay on target and not get lost in that way.

Most of us do not even know that many times a day they slip into this state of hypnosis. This can happen while you enjoy a book, play a computer game or just do a job. This state allows you to narrow your concentration and enhance your brain's processing of information. The ultimate objective of self-hypnosis is to establish a point of access to the part of your brain (subconscious) that regulates your emotions, habits or behaviors.

2 Simple Steps to Success with Self-Hypnosis

Try and think of your younger days, see if you can recall how easy it was to concentrate on certain things with all of the noisy humdrum that you are now older. It is a common belief that with the aging of our intelligence, but if you consider how many vital abilities we learn quickly in our early lives, this belief can be questionable.

Through self-hypnotism, the unconscious can be retrained and the ability to learn new complex skills as an adult can seem previously unlikely. The unconsciousness is what forms the personality and psychologically drives you.

Techniques of hypnotism have come a long way since yesterday's spinning pocket watch. Self-hypnosis is now a very valid way for us to get rid of the personality characteristics that may annoy us. Things like shyness, lack of confidence, excessive consumption, and smoking cigarettes can all be overcome by focusing on themselves.

Your willingness to accept the procedure depends on the success of self-hypnosis. The hypnotization process is really just two simple steps.

Step 1-Total relaxation is required.

You have to put yourself in a sleep state. Do not sleep as you go to bed at night, unconsciously and deliberately, but in a trance-like state. This can be achieved by lying or sitting in a quiet place and counting between 20 and

Concentrate on your breathing and you will relax with each exhale. Once you are relaxed, move on to step 2.

Step 2-Concentrate on a sentence or suggestion to achieve the objective.

You will be in a higher concentration than in normal thinking mode. All five of your senses are in a hyper-conscious state. Your proposal should be positive in context and repeated time and time again in order to integrate it into your subconscious. You will most probably experience rapid movement of the eye, REM.

This does not indicate that you are asleep because unlike normal sleep, you can wake up when you wish with self-hypnosis.

If you want to use self-hypnosis as a method to alter things in your life, you have to allow your desire to make you surrender. Your unconscious will build the initial momentum to do something, but your conscious commitment is required to make the big changes of your thought.

In short hypnosis, willpower and determination are required.

CHAPTER 2

Introduction to Sleep

SLEEP AND THE IMPORTANCE OF SLEEP

Sleep is critical in the development of a person's learning skills and memory. According to research, when a person lacks sleep, he/she will find it difficult to focus. This will have a significant effect on his/her learning capabilities. It is also harder to consolidate memory when you are sleep-deprived, making it difficult for you to absorb and recall new information.

What will happen if you frequently get insufficient sleep? First of all, it can occur due to a variety of reasons, such as job-related, lifestyle, stress, or you simply have a hard time falling asleep. You have to learn how to solve the dilemma because not getting enough amount of sleep constantly can take a toll on your health in the long run.

Insufficient sleep causes health problems, but habitually sleeping for more than nine hours per day can also cause health issues. You must get sufficient rest that fits your age, health condition, and lifestyle.

Poor sleeping habits can lead to the following medical conditions:
1. Obesity. Some studies link lack of sleep to weight gain. It is proven that those who sleep eight hours a day have the lowest body mass index (BMI), while those who continuously get less than six hours of sleep get a higher than the average BMI. Lack of sleep, along with two other factors, such as overeating and lack of physical activities, can increase your risk of getting obese.

The body secretes hormones responsible for controlling a person's appetite, glucose, metabolism, and energy during sleep. When you don't get enough sleep, your system will increase its production of cortisol, also known as the stress hormone. This also prompts your body to create more insulin, a hormone that is responsible for the production of glucose and fat storage. When the body has a high amount of insulin, the tendency is to gain weight and be at risk of developing diabetes.

Lack of sleep is also a factor in why the body produces a low amount of leptin, the hormone responsible for giving signals to your brain that it already has enough food. It also leads to the system's production of too much ghrelin, a biochemical that will always make you hungry and crave food. This is why it seems harder to satisfy your cravings when you lack sleep, and the kinds of foods you will crave are fattening, such as sweets. With your body feeling weak, you will no longer have enough energy to perform exercises that are needed to burn the excess calories you have taken.

2. Hypertension. Even when you only have trouble sleeping for one night, this can already worsen your existing hypertension problems. According to studies, having too little or too much sleep can increase the risk of a woman from developing coronary heart disease.
3. Diabetes. The body will find it challenging to process glucose when you lack sleep. Glucose is a kind of carbohydrate that serves as fuel for the cells. You are at a high risk of developing type 2 diabetes if this happens continuously.
4. Mood disorder. A person's mood is profoundly affected when he/she lacks sleep. The tendency is to get irritable and moody. If you allow this to happen all the time, it can lead to worse conditions, such as anxiety, depression, and mental distress. Several studies have shown how people's moods are affected by lack of sleep. The results include feeling low and pessimistic, quickly getting angry and sad. There are also a lot of subjects who felt mentally drained after losing precious hours of sleep. All these symptoms rapidly disappear, and the subjects feel better after getting back to their regular sleeping routine.
5. Alcohol dependency. There is a higher chance of getting dependent on alcoholic drinks when you often lack sleep.

Alcohol serves as a mild sedative. It is used by those who have insomnia to make it easier for them to sleep. Instead of providing a solution, this only worsens the problem. The effects of alcohol are temporary. The body will finish processing the alcohol after a few hours, which will alert and stimulate parts of your brain. This will wake you up and make it hard to go back to sleep.

If you are insomniac or have other problems that lead to poor sleep quality, you must find other solutions and not get dependent on alcohol.

With so many adverse effects of insufficient sleep on a person's health, it is believed that the problem is linked to lower life expectancy. Do not wait until it is already too late. Having sufficient and quality sleep has many benefits. Find solutions to your problem and find out about the available treatment options to make it easier for you to fall into a deep slumber.

Health Benefits of Sleep

Confident people tend to ignore the benefits of having a night of adequate sleep. For them, it is only part of the usual routine. If you look into the matter deeply, you are lucky if you don't have any trouble sleeping.

Fallowing a healthy sleeping habit affects your body in a variety of ways and causes the following health benefits:

1. Longer lifespan. Aside from making you healthier, having sufficient sleep affects the quality of your life. It makes you feel better and gives you a lighter aura to how you will go about your daily routine. Upon waking up, you will feel refreshed and energized, which is the opposite when you lack sleep, or you overslept.
2. Better memory. Your mind works as you sleep. It consolidates the skills that you have learned during your waking hours.

    For example, you are trying to learn a new language. Your mind will help you retain the information as you sleep. Upon waking up, it is easier to remember the words that you have already encountered, continue the learning process, and memorize more unfamiliar words and phrases faster.

Aside from consolidating memories, your brain also restructures or reorganizes as you sleep. This will help spur your creativity or form ideas, especially if you are thinking about what to paint, draw, or write. Studies have found that the emotional factors of a person's memory are strengthened by having a sufficient amount of sleep. It is what ignites your creative blood and ideas upon waking up.

3. Perform better at school. In 2010, the Journal Sleep found out that children aged 10-16, who suffer from interrupted breathing, such as sleep apnea and snoring, are more prone to having difficulties in learning and focusing. This had a significant effect on how they performed in school. It is okay to sacrifice sleep once in a while, but make sure not to do it all the time. Lack of sleep has opposite effects on adults and kids. Adults tend to lose energy and feel sleepy. Kids show symptoms that are similar to those who are suffering from ADHD. Kids who lack sleep are more likely to get hyperactive, impulsive, and inattentive.
4. Reduce the risk of having inflammation. People who get less than six hours of sleep at night tend to have higher blood levels of proteins that cause inflammation as compared to those who get sufficient rest. When this happens, you are placing yourself at a high risk of developing diseases, such as diabetes, stroke, heart problems, and arthritis. This will also affect your appearance and will make you look older at a faster rate.
5. Decrease your stress levels. It is only natural to face various stressful factors in your everyday life. Higher stress level makes you susceptible to cardiovascular diseases. There are many ways to battle out stress, and one of the most effective techniques is to sleep and get sufficient rest. It will clear your mind and give you a refreshed outlook. This way, you will have an easier time facing your troubles and thinking of how to counter these.
6. Improved performance for athletes. Having a sufficient amount of rest will boost your stamina, which is essential when you are involved in physically draining activities. This will make you a better athlete because you can move with more confidence and will not quickly get fatigued. It is a requirement for those who are involved in sports, such as football, tennis, and swimming.
7. Healthy weight. If you are planning to lose weight, make sure that you get sufficient sleep. Many dieters feel hungrier when

they lose sleep. This is because the same sectors of the brain control sleep and metabolism.
8. Happier mood. Lack of sleep can make you feel moody. Enough rest makes your emotions more stable, decreases your anxiety, and makes you feel more comfortable. It helps improve your mood so that you don't get irritated and angry easily. No matter how busy you are, you need to find a balance and get enough rest every day. If you sleep too much during the weekends, it means you aren't getting sufficient rest during the week. This is not healthy. You cannot make up for lost sleep by sleeping too much for a day or two.
9. Healthy skin. During the first three hours of your deep slumber, the body is most active in producing growth hormone, which is essential in the skin repair process. The next two hours are the phase when rapid eye movement (REM) begins. It is when the body produces melatonin, a kind of hormone that acts as an antioxidant. Most REM sleep happens during the last three hours. It is when the skin's temperature reaches its lowest, causing the muscles to relax and allowing the skin to recover. You need to experience each phase every night as you sleep, so your skin needs at least nine hours of sleep to become healthier.
10. Stronger immune system. Some studies proved that people who slept adequately are less likely to get sick compared to those who frequently lose sleep.
11. Lower risk of injury. Many reported accidents happened due to drivers who fell asleep or were sleepy while on the road. In the US alone, it is estimated that one out of five car accidents that happen in a day is caused by drowsy driving. There are many other kinds of accidents that you can avoid if you are alert because you've got enough rest. These mishaps include falling, slipping, accidentally cutting yourself, and many more.

12. Better sex life. Men who often get insufficient sleep have lower testosterone levels than those who follow a healthy sleeping routine. Your sex life will also likely suffer because you are quite tired due to a lack of sleep. It is worse when you are only on the dating level and often fall asleep during a movie or look uninterested while having a dinner date. It all boils down to balance. No matter how busy you are, you must always remind yourself that sleep is essential.

HEALTHY SLEEP – WHAT YOU NEED TO KNOW

Turning night into day is of little use. Of course, each person's need for sleep is an individual matter. Nevertheless, in this critical process for us, one can always distinguish the special phases of rest in a state of deep and shallow sleep. The data of the so-called architecture of sleep indicates that in the first half of the night, we are mostly in a deep sleep, while the second we spend more time in light, shallow sleep, or in a state of slumber.

Dive-In Dream

The essence of the process of falling asleep can be understood by the example of the image of focusing our internal energies or attention. Everyone knows from experience how it can tire, for instance, from reading. Shortly before the eyes begin to close, consciousness in a unique way narrow. The gaze freezes, the meaning of the writing starts to slip away, as the reader has already plunged into deeper spheres. Finally, he falls asleep.

We can say that falling asleep is nothing more than immersion in a trance. Everyone has this ability, and even before birth because the fetus is already sleeping in the mother's body. There are various aids and strategies to achieve this trance state quickly. Following the processes outlined, you relax fully, and external factors will have the least influence on your sleep pattern.

What Happens When We Finally Go to Sleep? Where Does Our Consciousness Go?

As for consciousness, perhaps the most reliable results in its study have been achieved where they have been interested in these issues for hundreds, if not thousands, of years: in the East with its developed Hindu and Buddhist traditions. They start from the fact that there is some kind of comprehensive consciousness, which Buddhists describe as "Buddha consciousness." One who wakes up (i.e., learns to maintain self-consciousness) to this level of consciousness will recognize and know everything in this world as inseparable and interconnected.

It seems that we are all closest to this state in the phase of deep night sleep. If we could maintain clarity of consciousness at this time, we would already be in a state of genuine bliss. Buddhist Zen masters and other people state that in this sea of deepest peace, at the very depth of consciousness, there is an incredibly powerful energy of development and healing. This energy allows you to look at the phase of deep sleep in a completely new, incomparably more significant light.

Considering this phase of sleep, representatives of scientific knowledge lose sight of the fact that during it, there is a release of the most significant amount of growth hormone. This explains why we should not deprive ourselves of the deep sleep phase, as well as why this phase occurs primarily in the first half of the night.

The Phases of Rest and Activity

Recording with the help of an electroencephalograph of typical samples of brain waves allows us to explain the phenomenon of relaxation states. The first half of night sleep primarily serves as a body regeneration (deep sleep), the second - the sensory, spiritual integration of the body (BDG-dream).

Researchers make even more specific differences and distinguish four phases of consciousness and regeneration induced by the human brain. In the phase of falling asleep, relatively chaotic beta waves (13-30 Hz) of waking consciousness give way to calmer alpha waves (8-12 Hz). Behind them come even slower theta waves (4-7 Hz), and finally, delta waves (1- 3 Hz), indicating the arrival of deep sleep. In general, we go from four to five phases of sleep for every hour and a half. This way of traveling "through the valleys and along the hills" reflects the fundamental picture of our night's rest. An individual "sleep profile" always has these characteristics.

During a night's sleep, the described rhythms continue to take place; only the consequences follow from them. If the alarm clock rings when a person is in a deep sleep, he gets up with a feeling of brokenness.

Sleep Regulators

Sleep is controlled by a specific kind of internal clock that is "located" in the brain and sets the rhythm of sleep and wakefulness. This rhythm does not allow itself to be changed, even if such an impression is created in case of sleep disturbance.

How Long Should You Sleep?

Concerning the question of how much a person needs to sleep, several theories are supported by more and more scientific facts. In principle, people can be typified by their need for sleep, as well as, for example, by the type of food.

Most people feel best after seven to eight hours of sleep. Studies show that many fail to oversleep at this much-needed time. In the morning, the alarm clock pulls them out of a nap before the body wakes up naturally. Many feel unwell if they manage to sleep for less than six hours. Several studies suggest that ten hours of sleep is the upper limit; sleep longer than that for an adult is already unreasonable.

It seems that children need ten to eleven hours of sleep, while they can also be classified into different types according to their need for sleep. It is possible that a relatively short night's rest and several sleep breaks during the day, the duration of which would be an average of half an hour, in their combination are ideal for many people.

Sleep Quality

If we talk about the quality of sleep, then we should touch on such a favorite topic as sleep until midnight. It has been said about this that it is unusually refreshing and invigorating, and classical medicine for a long time only laughed at these allegations. However, evidence-based medical facts appeared that reinforced the truth of ancient knowledge.

At about three in the morning, the development of growth hormone, which plays a crucial role in the realization of many regenerative possibilities of sleep bordering on a miracle, ends. From three o'clock, the hormonal restructuring of the body from night to day begins. Already at this early hour, the mechanism of cortisone production is activated, which is primarily responsible for the feeling of anxiety and activity, and these states are aimed at counteracting the body's stress factors.

On the contrary, hormonal sources of regeneration and renewal work most intensively during early sleep until midnight. Interestingly, this applies equally to "owls" and "larks." So, "owls," having switched to a different regime, can bring substantial benefits to their body.

Experience in implementing the concept of so-called daytime sleep supports this assumption. Those who go to bed at eight in the evening require much less sleep to achieve the same therapeutic effects. Soon after midnight, they again become vigorous and get at their disposal a lot of time to do their daily work at night. The explanation for this phenomenon lies in the natural, proven over millions of years of rhythm, which is normal. It has its advantages.

In ancient times, a man built his life, focusing on natural rhythms, which is still done by all animals living in the wild, as well as archaic nationalities. Anyone who is trained to think by analogy and realizes what natural rhythms are will understand that natural sleep has undoubted advantages and has not lost its relevance in nature to this day. True, in the life of a modern person, he often brings social problems.

Fixing Your "Organic Clock"

Another essential recommendation regarding the quality of sleep, we can derive from the ancient Chinese doctrine of the laws of bodily functions, the so-called organic clock.

According to this teaching, at eight o'clock in the evening, the segment of the day begins when the curve of sexuality and blood circulation is at its zenith. So, this time is ideal for going to bed, not just to fall asleep, but to sleep with a partner. Ten in the evening is the time to start the activation of the triple heater, that is, the time of intensive energy exchange, which is even more suitable, for example, for the holidays of love. This time continues until midnight.

After midnight, at the hour of spirits, the period of the gallbladder begins, and after it (until four in the morning) comes the time of the liver. In these early hours, the body can safely digest and remove toxins. Just at this time, most people are sleeping.

Four o'clock in the morning is the beginning of lung activation, in the Indian yogic tradition at this time it is prescribed to practice breathing practices (pranayama).

From six in the morning, the large intestine is maximally activated, in favor of which the early onset of stool in many people testifies. From eight o'clock in the morning, the stomach takes over the watch, requiring a filling.

Adherents of natural sleep find in these facts a logical confirmation of the loyalty of their chosen path; however, their opponents too...

If we also take into account the achievements of modern chronobiology, it will be possible to draw exciting conclusions, from which the higher and lower points of activity of the natural activity of the whole organism will become evident. So, the morning is a time of slow beginning. Muscles and joints are still in a stale state. Anyone who gives themselves an excessive load during these hours weakens the immune system and creates stress for the heart, as evidenced by the results of a British study involving swimmers. In the morning, the metabolism is at its zenith, which can be regarded as a scientific justification for the idea: "Have breakfast like a king."

From seven to eight o'clock in the morning, the body activating the "stress" hormones adrenaline and norepinephrine are produced in increased quantities. This enables the mechanism of fat breakdown in cells, which contributes to the assimilation of incoming food. In lying on the bed at this time, which is so loved by many dormice, there is not enough sense and logic.

Ideally, from noon to three in the afternoon, you should only deal with routine affairs, because at this time, the intensity of making mistakes is very high, and working capacity, on the contrary, is very modest. From three until seven in the evening, our long-term memory is in the phase of the highest activity, so that "headwork" training during these hours is more than appropriate and brings the best results. As for the owls, this rhythm can have a two-hour correction, and the corresponding period can last up to nine in the evening.

The time from seven to eleven in the evening is a time of feelings and sensuality. The heart rate slows, blood pressure decreases, body reactions become calmer, we feel more relaxed. All this creates a peaceful mood in a person. Therefore, this time is well suited for conversations and emotional contact. By the way, eating during these hours can be especially satisfying, although several facts are more likely against late dinners.

At the same time, you can look at the lifestyle of the population of the Mediterranean countries. Their inhabitants celebrate the end of the day and, at the same time, are rightfully among the healthiest nations in the world. When else can you afford a glass of wine, if not during the period of maximum activity of the senses?

WHAT KIND OF A SLEEPER ARE YOU?

Have you ever sat in a car or bus in a traffic jam and looked around at the other drivers and passengers? Have you noticed how many of them are yawning, looking stressed to the eyeballs and only half awake? It's all too common these days. Poor sleep, poor diet, lack of exercise, way too much stress and constant pressure. No wonder the number of prescriptions for sleeping pills and depression is increasing. But our mission is to do something practical to address this problem. It's time for action!

Sleep is the most precious restorative that rights so many physical and mental wrongs. It's the sweet elixir that transforms life and puts a spring in your step, a smile on your face and the feeling that you can take care of everything that comes your way. Sleep. Undervalued, ignored and forgotten until you wake up to the realization that it's one of the essential foundations of a profound sense of well-being.

So, what kind of a sleeper are you? There are many studies and descriptions of how we sleep but the common consensus settles for the following five simple categories:

Lively, Healthy Early Risers!

These happy individuals usually get all the sleep they need and rarely feel exhausted or fatigued. They are typically younger than the other groups, usually married or with a long-term partner, working full-time and definitely a morning person with no serious medical conditions.

Relaxed And Retired Seniors

This is the oldest group in the survey with half of the sample being 65 or older. They sleep the most with an average of 7.3 hours per night compared to 6.8 across all groups. Sleep disorders are rare even though there is a significant proportion with at least one medical disorder.

Dozing Drones

These busy people are usually married/partnered and employed but they often work much longer than forty hours a week. Frequently working up to the hour when they go to bed, they get up early so they're always short of sleep and struggle to keep up with the daily pressures of life. Statistically, they'll feel tired or fatigued at least three days a week.

Galley Slaves

This group works the longest hours and often suffers from weight problems as well as an unhealthy reliance on caffeine or energy drinks to get through the day. Shift workers often fall into this group and there is also a marked tendency to be a night owl or an evening person. They get the least amount of sleep of all and are more likely to take naps yet, surprisingly, this group often believes that, despite the state of their health, they are getting enough sleep.

Insomniacs

Here we can find the largest proportion of night people and many of them quite rightly believe they have a sleep problem. About half of this group feel they get less sleep than they need, and the same proportion admits to feeling tired, fatigued and lacking energy most of the time.

So, which of the five groups do you think you fit into?

If you're a fortunate member of Group One, your sleep should by definition be absolutely fine. But don't worry. The book's advice takes your needs into account too. We've got some really good ideas to share with you to help you keep on track and we'll even add some special extra features to your nightly rest routine to maximize the experience. If you're not in this group, our aim is to help you become a full-time member of the healthy, happy sleepers' association! Membership is for life.

The second group also tends to sleep pretty well but we have some great tips to improve the overall quality of your sleep and your health and make sure you always maximize the benefits of a good night's rest.

Group Three represents too many tired, irritable and generally inefficient individuals whose quality of life is impaired because they're too tired too often. Their work suffers because they rarely have sufficient rest to assimilate the day's events successfully. Their home life is degraded because work intrudes too often and they're just too tired to enjoy the pleasures and comfort of a life away from work. Feeling tired becomes their default position and they know they need to do something to give their minds and bodies the rest they need. Individuals in this group frequently suffer from long term mental, physical and emotional stress.

The fourth group is rightly described as the night owls. They work the longest hours and, as we noted above, they typically work shifts. The health problems associated with this group include a marked tendency towards obesity as well as a range of inflammatory diseases. Despite the fact that these people rarely look or feel well, they seem to ignore the evidence and usually claim to get enough sleep, relying on sugary energy drinks and caffeine to keep them awake during waking hours. They take naps because their bodies can't function without additional sleep during the day. An objective analysis of their health would typically reveal a range of health and well-being issues.

Insomniacs are the dominant members of Group Five, people who don't get enough sleep, can't get to sleep and who usually recognize that they have a problem. Unfortunately, many insomniacs end up taking prescription medication to deal with their symptoms and we have to question the benefits of this solution in the light of the many unpleasant side effects associated with long-term sleeping pill dependency. For insomniacs, life is a constant struggle because of the accumulative effects of long-term sleep deprivation.

EFFECTS OF SLEEP DEPRIVATION ON YOUR BODY

A poor sleeping habit has been linked with several health problems by science. His sufferings vary from gaining weight to a feeble immune system.

You know exactly how it feels when you are unable to sleep at night, spending the night turning and tossing on your bed - cranky, out of sorts and tired. But missing those nine hours of sleep can do more harm to your body than just making you feel grumpy. You may be unaware of the serious consequences that sleep loss can lead to, but they are real.

Here are the surprising and severe impacts that sleep loss can have on your body.

The internal systems of your body interfere with chronic sleep deprivation.

Central Nervous System

It is the pathway that helps in the transfer of all the crucial information of your body. Sleep is the key that helps the system to function in an orderly manner.

This flow of information can easily get disrupted when a person has chronic insomnia. It is while we are asleep that connections are formed between the neurons inside our brain that help us to remember the information we have learned. Your brain gets exhausted because of sleep deprivation and cannot perform its functions as a result.

The transmission of signals by your body may also get delayed, thus decreasing the coordination, increasing the danger of accidents, and decreasing your concentration levels.

Mood swings and compromised decision-making methods are the negative side effects of not giving enough rest to your body.

Respiratory System

Sleep loss can have direct impacts on your respiratory system. A possibly serious sleeping illness, obstructive sleep apnea, repeatedly causes discontinuous breathing during sleep. As you were awake for the whole night, you were deprived of the proper sleep and made you more vulnerable to infections like the flu and the common cold. Sleep deprivation can worsen any existing disease, for example, chronic lung illness.

Cardiovascular System

Your blood vessels and heart can function in a normal way only through certain processes that include blood pressure, inflammation levels, and blood sugar. These processes interfere with sleep loss. It is when you are asleep that your body repairs the blood vessels.

Cardiovascular diseases are found to be at their peak for people who do not give enough rest to their bodies. Moreover, insomnia has a connection with an increased danger of stroke and heart attack.

Immune System

A defensive, infection battling substance known as cytokines, is produced by your immune system when you are asleep. This substance is used by your immune system to combat foreign bodies such as viruses and bacteria and also helps you to sleep so that your system gets the time and energy to defend against diseases.

Sleep deprivation affects negatively by preventing the immune system from building up the forces and, thus, unable to ward off the invaders. It also might take a longer time to recover from the illness.

Digestive System

There are two hormones, ghrelin, and leptin, which are affected by sleep. Leptin gives instructions to your brain that you have eaten adequately, and you do not need to eat anymore. When you are unable to give yourself proper rest, leptin gets reduced, and the amount of ghrelin gets raised, which stimulates your appetite. The fluctuation in these two enzymes can increase your nighttime appetite.

Sleep deprivation also gives a hint to your brain to increase the levels of insulin after you have eaten. The greater amount of insulin in your blood can cause type II diabetes and promote the storage of fat.

Sleepiness Leads to Forgetfulness

In the year of 2009, some researchers from France and America performed experiments where they determined certain events of the brain, which were called "sharp wave ripples." These are the oscillatory arrangements in the brain of mammals that are seen when the brain is at rest, specifically during sleep. These arrangements are responsible for strengthening one's memory. The recent data that has been learned is transferred by the ripples to the neocortex from the hippocampus inside the brain. The neocortex is the region used for storing long-term thoughts. These ripples are known to occur when a person is in deep sleep.

Sleepiness Leads to Depression

Sleeping disorders are the main cause of depression. In 2005, a sleeping poll was conducted in America, where people who were identified to have depression were the ones who got six or even fewer hours of sleep at night.

Insomnia has got the strongest link with depression. It is rather the first symptom of anxiety. Both are related to each other. Depression can make a person not sleep at night, and sleep loss can provoke depression. But there is also a positive side to it. Treating depression can improve your sleeping habits and vice versa.

Sleep Loss Makes You Look Aged

Not getting enough rest is the main reason why some of us get dark circles, fine lines, and skin that lacks luster. It makes us look aged even when we haven't crossed the line of thirty.

Cortisol is released when we are in excessively stressed-out situations. This stress hormone, in its excess amount, is responsible for breaking down the protein found in skin, known as collagen, which is beneficial for our skin. It helps to keep your skin smooth and increases elasticity.

The growth hormone in human beings is released when we are asleep, and its amount can be reduced due to sleep loss.

Sleep Deprivation and Death Rate

Sleep patterns were found to have a great impact on the mortality rate of humans. Based on a result that was published in the year of 2007, it was proved that the risk of death was increased for a person who had cut down their sleep from nine to five hours and those with irregular sleep schedules. Death risks from cardiovascular disease have doubled with a decreased quantity of sleep. Serious circumstances like fatal familial insomnia, although in rare cases, can cause your death.

How Much Sleep Do We Want?

The Majority of us Need 8 hours of sleep per night to work properly approximately -- but a few want more and less. What's that you attempt to reach it and discover how much sleep you want.

As a general rule, in case you wake up exhausted and devote the day longing to get an opportunity to have a rest, probably, you are not obtaining sufficient sleep.

What Happens If I Do Not Sleep?

An Intermittent night with no sleep makes you feel irritable and tired the following day, but it will not damage your wellbeing.

After The effects, sleepless nights. Your mind will fog, which makes it hard to focus and make decisions. You might fall asleep and begin to feel down. Your risk of accidents and harm in the home and about the street raises.

In case it continues, insufficient sleep can affect your health and also make you prone to health conditions, such as cardiovascular disease, obesity, higher blood pressure, and diabetes.

Here are seven Ways where a fantastic night's sleep can improve your wellbeing:

Sleep Promotes Immunity

Should you look, your pregnancy might be to blame, to catch every cold and flu that is going around. Absence of rest can interrupt your system, and that means you are unable to fend off germs.

Sleep Can Lean Down You

Sleeping Less may indicate that you put on weight! Various studies have demonstrated that they tend to get pressure and have a higher chance of becoming overweight.

It is considered to be since sleep-deprived individuals have decreased levels of leptin (the compound that makes you feel complete) and increased amounts of ghrelin (the hunger-stimulating hormone).

Sleep Promotes Mental Health

Given that A sleepless night can make you moody and irritable the day, it is not surprising that sleep may lead to stress and depression.

When people It was that many of them slept less than 6 hours, with depression or anxiety surveyed to figure their habits.

Sleep Prevents Diabetes

Studies Have suggested that they have an elevated chance of diabetes. It sounds by merely altering the way that overlooking heavy sleep can lead.

Sleep Increases Libido

Men possess not as much interest in sexual activity and desires, the study indicates.

Sleep Wards Off Heart Disease

Long-standing Sleep deprivation appears to be associated with a higher heart rate, a rise in blood pressure, and more excellent rates of the specific substances related to inflammation, which might place additional strain on your heart.

Sleep Raises Infertility

Difficulty conceiving a baby maintained as one of the consequences of sleep deprivation in women and men. Sleep disruptions may lead to trouble by reducing the secretion of tissues conceiving.

The way to catch up on lost sleep.

Should you do not get enough sleep, there is just one way to compensate.

It won't occur with a single night. If you have had months of limited sleep, then you will have built up a substantial sleep debt, therefore expect the recovery to take a few weeks.

Beginning on Per night, A weekend, then try to include on an additional hour or two of sleep. The means to do so is to go to bed if you are tired and enable your body to wake you in the daytime (no alarm clocks!).

Expect to Sleep, in the beginning, every night for up to 10 hours. After a time, the quantity will fall to a degree.

Do not rely on energy or caffeine drinks as a soft drink. They can boost concentration and your power but may interrupt your sleep patterns much farther.

How to Attain an Absence of Deep Sleep

Almost everyone can reap the benefits of getting more sleep, and sleep looks more desirable. A lack of sleep can have severe health effects. Precisely what constitutes "deep" sleep, and also just how can you decide if you are getting enough of it? If you are not, and what achieved?

Deep sleep Describes the phase of sleep slow-wave rest, and also the somebody. Characterized by electrical activity in the brain's frontal lobes, it happens more. It's occasionally referred to as sleep or 4 phase 3 which also contains what was formerly called stage 4 sleep.

The 4 Stages of Sleep (NREM and REM Sleep Cycles)

Kids have more quantities of sleep. Compared to men, sleep is experienced by women during their lifetimes. In the study, research demonstrated while the proportions of women improved, the slow-wave rest of men diminished with age. Between ages 37 and 54, guys had a mean of 11.2% slow-wave sleep, and girls had 14.2%. Past age 70, the gap increased to 5.5% in males and 17.2% in girls.

Health Benefits of Deep Sleep

During heavy Sleep, the body releases hormones necessary for repair and the growth of cells. It's of critical importance for healthy development during childhood. It has a continuing part in adults, developing muscle mass with exercise, and relieving the effects of normal wear and tear in the human body. The blood circulation into the muscles.

Sleep may have roles in Preventing metabolic waste in mind through the circulatory system (such as a protein known as beta-amyloid). It maximizes system function, enhances memory processing and integration, and restores mobile energy stores.

How to Decide Whether You're Getting Enough Deep Sleep

The thickness Sleep can correspond to its quality--when you aren't getting enough sleep, you can tell. Mild sleep may be fragmented, punctuated by frequent arousals (alterations from heavy to light sleep) or awakenings. You might feel unrested and expertise sleepiness and fatigue throughout the day when you awaken.

Regrettably, Currently, there isn't any accurate and effortless method to quantify your sleep phases and determine whether you're getting enough sleep on a nightly basis. The standard gold evaluation for sleep investigation is that the polysomnogram, formal research done at a sleep center that steps:

The electric activity of the mind (and, by extension, sleep phases) having an EEG.

Muscle Action from the chin Eye movements

Breathing patterns Oxygen Amounts

The center Rhythm has an electrocardiogram (ECG or EKG) Leg movement.

This Testing has limitations since it's oblivious with sleep tracking preoccupied to sleep costly and inaccessible. Even though it's highly accurate at determining the existence and quantity of heavy sleep, it isn't helpful at all to somebody who introspectively wants to evaluate their sleep.

Wearable Technology, such as physical fitness trackers and apparatus that are related, seems to provide the promise of long-term and advantage evaluation. These devices are highly resolute by the detection of motion, heart rate, and occasionally other factors like oxygen levels or perhaps EEG. All these are incomplete surrogates for heavy sleep's hallmarks. Improvements from the science supporting the health technology may improve the accuracy of these dimensions. It may give us a means every evening to know the depth of their sleep experience.

Reasons for Deficiency of Deep Sleep

Consider These possible contributors to a lack of sleep:

Weakened Sleep push: Sleep diminished, and the ratio of heavy sleep decreased by taking fractures or even spending a protracted period in bed to the stage that there is no longer the inherent ability to sleep soundly.

Sleep Ailments: profound sleep may disturb. These disruptions may reduce the rest. Treatment can make a rebound of sleep and normalization of sleep stages' equilibrium.

Substance Withdrawal and use: Caffeine is a stimulant that reduces sleep. It might have impact hours. Likewise, rest is reduced by the use of drugs. (Conversely, withdrawal in the benzodiazepine medicine appears to improve deep sleep.) An antidepressant that's frequently working as a sleeping aid, trazodone, seems to enhance sleep through impacts on the system that is histamine. Both lithium and marijuana, a medicine for bipolar illness, may improve sleep.

Boost sleep Drive: prolonged periods of strengthening what referred to as raising the nap as the sleep drive. That if you do get to bed, then you achieve sleep, to put it differently, you might have to decrease the chance for rest. Sleep consolidation, or sleep restriction, is an excellent remedy for insomnia that's incorporated into cognitive-behavioral treatment for insomnia (CBTI) program. When sleep happens, sleep deprivation may improve sleep depth.

Adhering to a Circadian rhythm sleep follows a circadian pattern. It could be better by visiting a standard sleep-wake program, such as on weekends, and utilizing morning sunshine as a constant cue into the circadian rhythms immediately upon waking when sleeping is intermittent, summary by deep sleep's time.

Behaviors and surroundings study are required to comprehend the ramifications of the situation and clinics about maintenance and the initiation of sleep. Exercise and decent daylight physical activity may assist, but the perfect timing is not as precise. Taking a bath or shower for around 90 minutes can help with sleep's start. There's some evidence that a bedroom temperature enhances sleep. Light or surround sound, or an elevated temperature, can endanger it. It's also possible that external apparatus -- such as those who emit varying electric patterns, sounds, vibrations, or mild --might have a part in improving sleep thickness.

Hazards Related to Lack of Deep Sleep

There are Clear signs that a lack of sleep has consequences on health. The quality of sleep plummets when sleep is compromised. As mentioned above, there may be the mind, effects on the human body also, notably. Consider these effects:

Pain: Decreased sleep exacerbates pain. It can manifest in a variety of ways, such as a diagnosis of fibromyalgia. Pain can decrease as sleep thickness enhances.

Impaired Development: Kids that suffer from obstructive sleep disorders like sleep apnea encounter diminished sleep. It impairs the release of growth hormones. Luckily, once handled, a growth rally experienced by these kids.

Dementia: The accumulation of plaques inside brain tissue disrupts the maturation of Alzheimer's disease and memory impairment. A lack of sleep, that is, and the disturbance of the practice of cleansing the mind of the proteins, may hasten this illness.

If you're worried about a reduction of sleep, think about what is in your hands. Attempt to maximize the consistency of your program. Make a sleeping refuge, maintain the bedroom, and remove electronics that are disruptive. Avoid naps and guarantee you're not spending too much time trying to sleep (most adults need 7 to 9 hours of sleep to feel rested, but elderly adults might require 7 to 8 hours). Reduce caffeine intake and prevent chemicals that may reduce sleep. If you suspect you might have a sleep disorder like insomnia or sleep apnea, get assessed by a naturopathic sleep medicine physician. These modifications might be the secret to finishing a lack of sleep, boosting both health advantages and well-being.

HOW TO GET A GOOD NIGHT SLEEP

The effect of good night sleep cannot be overemphasized. It is primal to the mental, physical, and emotional wellbeing of a man. This explains why not getting adequate sleep does take its toll on physical wellbeing, productivity, and can even lead to excess weight. Unfortunately, due to the worries of everyday life, many people find it difficult to gather their thoughts and get a good night's sleep.

When you are wide awake at 2 am staring at the ceiling, getting a good night's sleep might seem like a mirage. The good news, however, is that you can take steps to control your sleep and ensure you get a good night's sleep. This can be traced to simple daytime routines that you overlook.

If you chose bad daytime habits like excess alcohol or exercise near the evening, it would surely affect your sleep. We, however, have some exciting tips with which you can get a good night's sleep.

Tip 1: Be in Tune with Your Sleep-Wake Cycle

One of the best strategies for getting a good night's sleep is being in sync with your circadian rhythm. If you maintain a definite sleep-wake cycle, the quality of your sleep will be better. Some tips to make this possible are:

Sleep at the same time every day

The idea behind this is to keep your body's internal clock regular, which will, in turn, boost the quality of your sleep. Your bedtime should be when you are stressed or tired. This will prevent you from turning and tossing.

Control Napping

We have no problem with napping, as it might be an excellent way to make up for a sleepless night. The issue with napping, however, is that it could affect the quality of your sleep at night. With this in mind, limit napping to a maximum of an hour in the early afternoon.

Control Urge to Sleep After Dinner

It is common and normal to feel sleepy after eating, especially if it is a heavy meal. Resist the urge to curl up your couch and sleep off. Rather, stand up and get moving. Find something to do, like doing the dishes, chatting with your spouse, reading, or pressing your clothes for the next day. Sleeping earlier than usual might make you wake up at midnight, leading to insomnia.

Tip 2: Be Smart with Light Exposure

There is a naturally occurring substance in the body called melatonin, which is controlled by light. The primary assignment is to regulate the sleep-wake cycle. In the dark, the brain secretes more melatonin, which induces sleep. In the light as well, the brain secretes less melatonin, which makes you pretty alert. The problem comes when the production of melatonin is altered. As a result, we will explore how to control your exposure to light.

Influencing Your Light Exposure During the Light

Get More bright light in the Morning: As early as possible every morning, get exposed to sunlight. Take a walk in your compound or swipe the blind so that light rays get inside.

Spend Enough Time Outside in the Day: when you have a work break, go for a walk. Exercise outside or take a walk with your dog.

Let in More Natural light into your office or Work. It is a good idea to have the window blinds open during the day at work or in your office.

Influencing Your light Exposure During the Night

Avoid Bright Screen an hour to Bed: The blue light coming from your mobile device, screen, TV, PC, etc. does not help your sleep. As a remedy, use light altering software or reduce the brightness totally if you cannot stay away from your gadgets.

Avoid Reading with Backlight Devices: Stop using phones, tablets, etc. to read at night.

Try and Sleep in a completely dark room: Keep light sources away from your room. Use a heavy curtain to block out light rays. Sleep with a mask if you cannot control the light source.

If you have to get out of bed at night, use dim lights. This will make it easy for you to fall back to sleep.

Tip 3: Exercise during the Day

Regular exercise is one of the best ways to get a good night's sleep. If you exercise during the day, you will sleep better at night. Regular exercise can help you beat insomnia. In addition, it also helps you dwell in a deep sleep more.

More vigorous exercise makes you sleep better at night. However, no matter how little they exercise, it will increase the quality of your sleep.

It is essential to build a quality exercise habit. This is because you might not see the effect of regular exercise until after a couple of months.

Be Smart with Your Exercise Timing

There are many benefits of exercise, such as increased body temperature, boosting heart rate, and increasing the rate of metabolism. This is nice if you exercise in the morning or afternoon. Exercising in the evening, however, can be a recipe for disaster.

With this in mind, your vigorous exercise should end in the afternoon. If you must exercise in the evening, make it low impact and gentle like yoga, stretching, or walking.

Tip 4: Take Note of What You Eat and Drink

Unknown to many, your choice of food also plays a pretty important role in influencing your sleep quality. As a result, keep the following in mind as they influence your diet:

Reduce Caffeine and Nicotine:

Unknown to many people, caffeine interferes with sleep. It can affect your sleep-in awful ways and could be active for as long as 12 hours after drinking it. Also, avoid smoking when it is near bedtime. It does not help your sleep.

Avoid Huge Meals at Night

Ideally, we recommend having your dinner early in the evening. It should be at least two hours before bed. A heavy meal will not help you. Stay away from spicy and acidic food as well.

Reduce Liquid Intake in the Evening

When you drink excess fluid, your bladder will be full, which will make you wake up incessantly to go to the bathroom. This affects your sleep.

Tip 5: Wind Down and Clear Your Head

There are many reasons people find it difficult to sleep well. It could be stress, anger, worry, anxiety, and many other factors. This is why you need to take steps to manage your mental health by reducing your overall stress level. It can go a long way in relaxing your mind and preparing you for a good night of restful sleep. The idea of this is to focus on developing helpful habits like relaxation techniques, meditations, listening to soft music, etc., intending to induce sleep.

If you find yourself bewildered with your worries such that it disturbs your sleep, you need to concentrate on this part. If you over-stimulate your brain during the day, settling down to sleep might be difficult. For instance, many people cannot focus on a single task for long. They are guilty of constantly looking for something new and fresh to stimulate themselves. This makes it pretty hard to relax.

The best way to go about this is to set extra time to relax, catch up with friends via chat, and check your social media. Also, the idea is to focus on a single task at once. This will help, and you will be able to calm your mind when you are about to sleep.

Sample Deep breathing Exercise to help Sleep better

The idea of this exercise is to make you breathe from your belly and not your chest. This way, you can activate relaxation techniques that will produce an instantaneous calming effect on your blood pressure, heart rate, and stress levels. The following steps discuss how to go about it:

Lay in a comfortable position with your eyes closed Have a hand on your chest and the other on your belly.

Breathe in through the nose and watch the hand on your belly rise. There should be a little movement with the hand on your chest.

Breathe out through your mouth and exhale as much air as you can. The hand on your belly should move in as you breathe in, while the other one should move a little

Keep repeating the cycle of breathing in and out through your nose and mouth. Suck in enough air to enable your lower abdomen to rise.

A Body Scan Exercise to help With Sleeping

When you direct your attention to various parts of your body, you can pinpoint anywhere that is tensed and take the needed steps to let go of it.

Lay down on your back with your legs spread out. Your eyes closed, and your arms by your side. Start breathing and direct your attention to it till you feel better.

Focus on your right toe. Look for any tension without directing your attention away from your breath. As you breathe, imagine each breath flowing from your toes. Keep your attention on your toes for at least three seconds.

Now focus on the sole of the same foot. Watch out for any sensation in that part of the body and imagine your breath flowing from the sole. Move your focus to the ankle, calf, knee, and other parts of the body. Spend more time on any body part that feels tense.

When you are done with the whole-body scan, take note of how the whole body feels. There should be a deep sense of relaxation that will make it easy to drift off.

HOW TO FALL ASLEEP, SLEEP, AND GET ENOUGH SLEEP

What You Need for Good Night's Sleep

Sleep disorders are difficult to tolerate, but this is not the only reason to do something to neutralize them. Sleep disorders shorten lifespan. They increase the risk of apoplexy, heart attack, and cancer. They make a person more susceptible to all kinds of infections, as they weaken the body's resistance. In addition, sleep dysfunctions increase the risk of accidents, and not only on highways. Those who sleep poorly do not die, but live, of course, much worse than they could.

Lying to Sleep, Only Feeling Tired

Body fatigue and spiritual fatigue are equally important for a good fall asleep. Physical work, walking, or sports - it doesn't matter how we get into a state of bodily fatigue. It is advisable that the corresponding activity is filled with subjective meaning. The same goes for spiritual fatigue. You should give yourself a constructive, meaningful load in order to promote your own development and the subsequent good fall asleep. If you still remain awake after fifteen minutes, try to get out of bed and stay on your feet until the feeling of "deadly fatigue" falls on you again, and you really don't want to go back to bed.

Fight for Good Sleep

Instead of balloting under the guise of diagnoses such as hypersomnia, or daytime sleepiness, or allowing you to diagnose such dysfunctions in yourself, it would be much more advisable to enter the fight for sleep with an open visor.

Anyone who can't sleep at night, and all day long only "bites his nose," has obvious problems in opening up to the dark time of the day and all the shadow gestalts hiding in it. So, his own subconscious mind tries to postpone the dream to "safer times."

However, such a dream, on the one hand, does not give the expected effect. On the other hand, he frustrates not only all plans for the day but also all kinds of social contacts. That is why it would be much more appropriate in the dark to face the dark aspects of being.

In such a situation, it is useful first of all to reveal your unconscious fear of darkness and its shadowy essences. Among the self-help programs that contribute to this are meditation and yoga.

The fight should also be waged at another level. Anyone who does not allow himself to give up fatigue throughout the day will sleep again sometime at night. The question arises: does the subconscious mind win, or does the consciousness continue to dominate? Snuggle against daytime sleepiness can take on a debilitating, destructive character, but, if necessary, a person can stand up if, while sitting, he cannot lose sleepiness. To those who make a firm decision not to sleep for a minute from nine in the morning until nine in the evening, and who are able to adhere to their plans, success will come quickly.

The likelihood of night sleep is high if the subconscious mind receives a message that it has no chance to compensate for the lack of sleep at any other time. We can always rely on the mind of our bodies.

Exercises

The key to quick and smooth falling asleep lies in the already mentioned action of liberating "from everything."

Those who unsuccessfully try to sleep, most likely, have not completely resolved a particular issue in the past, and this question, consciously or unconsciously, puts pressure and makes return to himself again and again. In such cases, it is advisable to do EC meditative exercises for a release.

High-quality sex with a bright orgasm in conclusion also contributes well to subsequent falling asleep. Orgasm, like a little death, clears the road to sleep.

Find Your Daily Rate

I can only let go of what I have dealt with. Of course, today's tasks have a complex structure and scope of events. And this stretches the process of solving them for days, weeks, or even months, and it is not possible to fully implement them within one day.

Anyone who self-critically assesses his ability to do a certain amount of work well enough for a certain time, and then sets himself this feasible goal, can introduce the concept of the daily rate of work into his life. Remember, we are able to do the intended amount of work but should not allow it to rule over us. Anyone who has accomplished a realistic task by the end of the day can complete the task with satisfaction. And then allow yourself peace - the peace that makes falling asleep for granted and a natural gift. Thus, a person returns to a state that during the previous millennia was completely normal.

In this way, all tasks can be divided into reasonable segments that can be dealt with during working hours. The simpler the task is structured, the easier it will be. If we are talking, say, about cleaning or ironing, about working in the garden or camping in the mountains, this is usually easy to do. Listed and similar activities allow you to relax and then plunge into a refreshing dream. But even in relation to modern, ambitious projects, it is useful to find a realistic individual daily rate of work and adhere to it.

Live in Rhythm

Sleep is one of human instincts. Nature has laid down certain rhythms in us: the rhythm of the seasons, the rhythm of day and night, and the rhythm of sleep and wake following from it. These rhythms form an elementary aspect of our life. They have tangible power over us, and it is far from easy to get out of them. The less we interfere in their course, the better. If we want to free ourselves from the yoke of sleep disorders, we need to return to our roots and do the correction of the disturbed rhythm of life.

In addition, the daily rhythm is a cast of a larger rhythm of our being. Recall that in the language, there are expressions about the zenith of life, that is, that segment of time when the vital forces (or the Sun) are at the highest point, as well as about old age as the sunset of life.

A lot of evidence suggests that people who have managed to return to the natural rhythm of life are cured of sleep disorders.

Sometimes during the long and dark winter months, when the difference between day and night is barely felt due to bleak weather conditions, despondency settles in the soul. The reason for this is to increase the concentration of the "night hormone" melatonin in the blood, and especially in the brain. At the same time, the concentration of the "hormone of happiness" serotonin is also reduced. Intensive light therapy using a special lamp can help. It has been proven that a certain amount of sunlight during the day is enough to normalize the lost rhythm of sleep and wakefulness.

In the normal case, a time under the sun or sunbath is enough for this. In the north and in our latitudes - in particular, during prolonged fogs - the absence of light can lead to symptoms of exhaustion.

It is strongly recommended that you maintain a stable rhythm of sleep and wakefulness throughout the days of the week. It is difficult for many people to sleep late at the weekend or to pick themselves up on the alarm clock on weekdays. They will be helped by a constant rhythm, which implies daily lifting and going to bed at the same time. If individually important sleep breaks are taken into account, this approach can bring good results.

Of course, there is a danger of becoming rigid or even stagnant in this regard. However, a return to a satisfactory sleep pattern is of primary importance at first. And at first, too rigid a regime can later turn into a life- giving rhythm - life-giving in the sense that it is determined in accordance with life and individual needs connected with it.

Analysis Matrix

The simplest sleeping pills can be extracted from such a course of action that does not exert active resistance to sleep. Previously, the motto of medicine was the motto: "Non nocere" ("Do no harm"). Each evening lesson should be viewed from that angle, whether it promotes sleep or prevents it.

If a person believes that he is no longer able to sleep at night (sleepy hypochondria), he should follow a double strategy. On the one hand, replenishment of the luggage of sleep knowledge can help (remember, in particular, the simple technique described in the heading "sleep disorder knockouts?", which involves putting down across every fifteen minutes during an allegedly sleepless night). On the other hand, one who understands the principle of the operation of self-fulfilling forecasts is not so easily caught by their bait.

On the whole, the realization of the principle of development of soul matrices is the first decisive step towards parting with them. Then a solution can be found at the same level. A state of deep relaxation, remember, is ideal for dealing with the root causes of anxiety and fear.

CHAPTER 3

Hypnosis Sessions for a Healthy Sleep

Disclaimer: when listening to hypnosis recordings, do so in a safe place, preferably where you will not be disturbed for the duration of your recording. Please use your headphones. Never listen to recordings or practice self-hypnosis while driving in a car, operating machinery, or doing anything else that requires your attention for safety reasons.

GENERAL RELAXATION SESSION

Before we begin, I'd like you to take a couple of minutes to prepare yourself for a restful sleep.

Prepare your room by turning off any devices that might be a distraction. You may need to put your phone in another room if you are tempted to check it repeatedly. Turn off the TV or any music that is playing. You want to set the stage for a night of rest and relaxation.

Dim the lights.

Lie down, on your back and settle into a position that is comfortable for you. If you are not comfortable lying on your back, you might want to put or rolled blanket under your knees. Make sure that your head and neck are supported as well.

If it is comfortable for you, try moving your head back and forth and turning it side to side to loosen up your neck muscles.

Let it relax back into a comfortable position.

Wiggle your shoulders and let them fall back into a relaxed position.

Keeping your buttocks on the bed, move your hips a bit and then let them fall back into a relaxed position.

You want your body to be in a neutral and comfortable position so:

Make sure that your chin is not pointing too far up. Tuck in just a bit to allow the neck to lengthen and the jaw to relax.

Tuck your shoulders underneath you and then let them relax into a natural position.

Let your hands rest at your sides, palms up or down, or on your abdomen.

Let your legs relax, your feet and knees may roll out when they are relaxed. Try not to hold them in any specific position, just let them fall naturally.

Pause to allow participants a couple minutes to adopt a comfortable position.

[Intention setting and focus on breathing: 10 minutes]

You may find that you will doze during this meditation. That is ok. Don't force yourself to stay awake if you feel that you are sleepy.

Close your eyes lightly. For this time, you aren't going to try to do anything. There is no need to worry about things that happened today or things that might happen tomorrow. Right now, all you need to do is to be here, in your body, on your bed letting your mind do what it needs to do to relax for a good night's sleep.

Thank yourself for taking this time for self-care. You deserve a night of restful sleep and to wake up feeling refreshed and ready for the day. This is one thing that you can do that is just for yourself. No guilt, no worries.

Know that whatever worries you and stops you from sleeping won't be fixed by keeping you awake.

Know that no matter how you slept last night, or the night before, you can sleep well tonight. This is the only night that matters.

Pause a minute for reflection.

During this meditation, each time you find your mind drifting, notice where it's gone and gently tell yourself to come back to being right here, right now. There is no need to judge what your mind is thinking about or that you have become distracted. This is what our brains are designed to do and most of us spend all day trying to think about many things all at once. It is not easy to undo years of training and it probably won't be undone today but you've already started doing the best thing that you can do to unclutter your mind.

Breath in and out naturally a few times.

Think about your breath but try not to change it. This is your natural breath. You do this all day without thinking about it. For just a few minutes, focus on this activity. So easy it happens without any thought or effort.

Pause a minute for reflection.

Take a few deep breaths and exhale whatever tension you feel. Inhale slowly and really feel where the air is going. It is normal to breath less than we can. Right at this moment, you want to breathe as fully as possible.

Take a deep breath and feel the air as it flows through your nostrils, down into your lungs and fully into your abdomen. Breathe in as deeply as you can.

Exhale slowly, pushing the air out, first from your abdomen and then from your lungs.

Think about any areas of tightness you may have had when you took that breath. If it felt stuck anywhere, feel what it would be like to relax in that area.

You are going to take a few deep breaths again and think about relaxing into the breath. I will be giving you instructions for relaxation but don't feel that you need to match the pace of your breath with my instructions. Just keep breathing deeply and try to apply the instructions with each breath.

When you exhale, don't push out the air so much that you are pulling in your stomach. Let the exhale come to a natural end with your body feeling relaxed and empty of air.

On your next deep inhale, feel the flow through your nostrils, down behind your jaw into your throat. Sometimes people tighten their throat when breathing deeply. Try to tuck your chin, just a bit, to lengthen your neck, relax your jaw and think about opening your throat to allow the air to pass freely through and into your lungs.

Exhale slowly, feeling the air flow out of your body. Pause a minute for reflection.

Inhale deeply again, feeling the air through your nostrils and throat and into your lungs. Relax your chest and let your lungs expand with breath. Think about opening your lungs out and not up. If you feel your shoulders rising, think about relaxing them back down and to the sides while letting your lungs push out with air.

Exhale fully and try that again. Inhale deeply into your lungs, relaxing your shoulder down and away from your ears and letting your lungs fill until they are large and full.

Exhale naturally.

Pause a minute for reflection.

On your next deep inhale, feel the airflow from your nostril, down your throat and into your lungs. Feel your abdomen rise as you fill your lungs. Relax your stomach and let it push out. Don't worry, no one is watching. Use your stomach to help your lungs fill more fully. A lot of us aren't used to relaxing our stomachs this way. We don't like to push it out and look fat but know that no one is watching you right now.

Exhale naturally, relax your stomach and try that again. Inhale deeply, feeling the air in your lungs and your abdomen pushing out. Relaxing your shoulders and letting your stomach push out.

Take three more deep breaths at your own pace, feel for any remaining areas of tension. Meet those areas without judgment and try to relax them. Don't worry if they still feel tight. Just take note of them as you move your attention elsewhere.

Let your breath relax and become natural again.

Pause a minute for reflection.

[Body scan: 10 minutes]

As your body relaxes, it may begin to feel heavy. Feel how it rests on the bed. You are supported in this meditation by the things around you. They hold you and allow you to do the work you need to do to unclutter your mind.

Like your breath, your body may hold areas of tension that distract you. As we scan the body, we will try to release these areas and achieve a fuller relaxation. When you notice tension, try to relax those muscles. You may find that a small stretch and release of the muscles helps reduce the tension. This doesn't have to be a big movement. It is something that resets the muscle memory into one of relaxation rather than tension.

Bring your attention to the top of your head. Focus on what that feels like. Maybe it's warm or maybe you feel a breeze. If you don't think about it much, it might be hard to feel the top of your head. Imagine it touching the air around you. You might feel something strongly, like heat or a breeze. Whatever you feel, or don't feel, is ok. Just notice whatever it is, without judgment.

Pause a minute for reflection.

Move your attention to your cheeks and around your mouth... Notice if you are holding tension in either of these places. Think about what to would feel like to let that tension go. Try bringing your lips into a soft small smile. This smile is mostly internal. It always feels better to smile and helps to relax your whole face. Don't worry if this all feels a little funny, just relax and let it happen or not without judgment.

Pause a minute for reflection.

Now bring your attention to your neck and shoulders. These are very common areas for storing stress and tension. If you keep them tight, you may not even be able to imagine what they would feel like relaxed. Try shrugging your shoulders and tucking them back. Move your head back and forth a little bit. If any of these actions hurts, stop. Let your shoulders feel heavy and fall away from your neck. Notice whatever you feel in your neck and shoulders without judgment. However much you relax them is more than they were relaxed before!

Pause a minute for reflection.

Focus on your heart area, stomach, and abdomen. Notice if you are holding any tension in those areas. Nerves and worries like to settle there. You can let those go for now. If you need them, they will come back But, for this small amount of time, you can just let them go. Thinking about your worries may have reminded you about something you need to start or finish (or start and finish). You have already promised yourself that you will get to those things when you are finished with this. You can let them wait for just a few more minutes while you prepare your mind for them. Holding tension in your stomach won't help them to get done. Try to imagine your chest and stomach relaxed and not distracting you from things you want to focus on.

Pause a minute for reflection.

Move your attention to your arms. They might feel heavy to you, that is how they are when they are relaxed. Let them rest however is comfortable for you. Notice if you have any tension in your hands and stretch your fingers just a bit to let that go. Let them relax again, resting on your legs or the floor.

Inhale

Exhale

Take one more deep breath and feel the weight of your body on the bed. This is rest. This is how you replenish.

Let yourself feel this fully and completely.

Let yourself rest.

GENTLE GUIDED SLEEP HYPNOSIS SESSION

If you feel any of these areas tensing up, focus your attention here. Breathe in... and breathe out... choose to relax and soften these areas. As you breathe, imagine the air bringing total relaxation to these areas and allowing the tension to leave your body. I invite you to continue this pattern until your breathing becomes deep and slow again.

Notice now how your body has become more relaxed than it was before. Feel your muscles sink into the bed as you relax further and deeper. Your jaw is becoming loose. Your mouth is resting, and your teeth are slightly apart. Now, your neck is relaxing, and your shoulders are falling away. Allow this to happen and let your muscles become soft.

I want you to return to your safe place. Imagine that this place is spacious, comfortable, and filled with a positive light. In this place, you have nothing to worry about, and you have all the time in the world to focus on yourself.

In this safe place, I want you to imagine the sun streaming in. The light fills you with warm and positive emotion. These are windows where you can see the beautiful nature outside. Your space can be wherever you want it to be. It can be by the mountains, by the ocean, or perhaps even on a golf course.

Return your focus back to your safe place. Imagine how warm and comfortable the room is. Walk over toward the comfortable bed and imagine how wonderful it feels to sink into the sheets. The sun is shining down on you, and you feel relaxed and warm. The bed is so soft around you, and you feel so at peace at this moment.

Notice now how these peaceful thoughts begin to fill your mind. They fill your consciousness and are clear. Any other thoughts you had before are drifting away. Your mind is falling into a positive place as you feel yourself drifting away. The space around you is safe and peaceful, and beautiful.

Any other thoughts you have at this moment pass through your mind and drift off like clouds drifting by. Allow these thoughts to pass without judgment. There is no sense in dwelling on them when you are in such a safe place. All you have at this moment is peace and quiet.

Any time a worried thought arises, you turn your focus back to your safe place. In this location, you can get rid of any stress you may have on a daily basis. You are here to relax and enjoy this moment. There is nothing that can bother you. You are free from stress and responsibilities here.

When you are ready, you feel your body begin to drift off to sleep. You are beginning to slip deeper and deeper toward the land of dreams. As you feel your attention drifting, you are becoming sleepier, but you chose to focus on counting with me. As we count, you will become more relaxed as each number passes through.

We will now take a few breaths, and then I will count from number one to number ten. As you relax, your mind will drift off to a deep and refreshing sleep. Ready?

Breathe in... one... two... three... and out... two... three.

Breathe in... one... two... three... and out... two... three.

Breathe in... one... two... three... and out... two... three.

Wonderful. Now, count slowly with me... one... bring your focus to the number one...

Two... you are feeling more relaxed ... you are calm and peaceful... you are drifting deeper and deeper toward a wonderful night of rest.

Three... gently feel as if all of the tension leaves your body. There is nothing but total relaxation filling your mind and your body. At this moment, your only focus is on quietly counting numbers with me.

Four... picture the number in your mind's eye. You are feeling even more relaxed and at peace. Your legs and arms are falling pleasantly heavy. You are so relaxed. Your body is ready to sleep.

Five... you are drifting deeper. Sleep begins to wash over you. You are at peace. You are safe. You are warm and comfortable.

Six... so relaxed...drifting off slowly...

Seven... your mind and body are completely at peace. You have not felt this calm in a while...

Eight... everything is pleasant. Your body feels heavy with sleep.

Nine... allow your mind to drift... everything is floating, and relaxing... your eyelids feel comfortable and heavy... your mind giving in to the thought of sleep.

Ten... you are completely relaxed, and at peace... soon, you will be drifting off to a deep and comfortable sleep.

Now that you are ready to sleep, I will now count from number one to number five. All I want you to do is listen gently to the words I am saying. When I say the number five, you will drift out of hypnosis and sleep comfortably through the night.

In the morning, you will wake up feeling well rested and stress-free. You have worked on many incredible skills during this session. You should be proud of the hard work you have put in. Now, it is time to sleep so you can wake up in the

SLEEP HYPNOSIS SESSION 1

Welcome.

This is going to be a thirty-minute guided hypnosis session to help you drift off into a deep and relaxing sleep. The most important thing to do while listening to this session is to keep an open mind. You must go with the flow, listen to my voice, and remember to breathe.

Remember, it is not always possible to enter a light hypnotic state on the first try, but we are going to try as I guide you gently and smoothly into this state so you can fall asleep. Please bear in mind that you are not going to enter any sort of deep catatonic state. Nothing is going to be physically altered within the realm of your mind. The process of hypnosis and this guided meditation is extremely safe, and you are in control of it.

Now, I want you to get comfortable. Because you are trying to achieve a deep sleep, you should be lying down, your head resting on your most comfortable pillow, and you are warmed by your softest blanket. Lie back and let your shoulders go slack, relaxing against the cushion of your bed. Gently close your eyes and release all the tension from your muscles. Release the tension in your arms, then your legs. Let go of the tension in your chest and in your back. All of the muscles in your body begin to feel looser and looser and your body is feeling light.

Focus your attention on your toes. Softly wiggle all ten toes once, and then again. Feel the energy released from your movement and the stillness that follows. Your toes are now ready for sleep.

Next, tighten the muscles in your calves and hold for one, two, or three seconds. Now release the muscles. Tighten them again for one, two, three seconds. Now release. The excess energy that keeps you up at night has been expelled from your calves. Your calves are now ready for sleep.

Next, squeeze your thigh muscles and hold for one, two, or three seconds. Now release. The tension that was once stored there has been released. Your thighs are now ready for sleep. Feel the lightness that has cloaked your legs. Your legs feel weightless as if they could float up to the ceiling.

Focus your attention on your buttocks. Tighten your muscles in buttocks for one, two, three seconds. Now release the muscles. The tightness in your buttocks and lower back has been relieved. Your buttocks and lower back are now ready for sleep.

Focus your attention on your abdomen. Squeeze your abdominal muscles for one, two, or three seconds. Now release. The anxiety that has been stored up and deterring sleep has been released. Your abdomen is now ready for sleep.

Concentrate on your chest. Tighten the muscles in your chest for one, two, three seconds. Now release. The sadness that has been weighing on you and preventing your mind from resting has been expelled. Your chest is now ready for sleep.

Direct your attention now to your shoulders. Tighten the muscles in your shoulder for one, two, three seconds. Now release. The stress that has been building in the deep tissue of your shoulders has now been dissolved. Your shoulders are now ready for sleep.

Focus your attention on your neck. Gently tighten the muscles and hold for one, two, or three seconds. Now release. Gently tighten the muscles in your jaw and hold for one, two, three seconds. Now release. Gently tighten the muscles in your mouth and hold for one, two, or three seconds. Now release. Gently squeeze your eyelids tighter for one, two, or three seconds. Now release. The tension that was held in your face has now been released.

The entirety of your body has been washed with serenity as you expel the negative energy from your muscles. Now that your body is relaxed, your mind can now relax in preparation for deep slumber. Realize how free it feels to let go of all built up tension. In this moment nothing else matters. You are free. You are relaxed. You are weightless.

There is nowhere for you to be, and you have everything you need. You are here, in this moment, permitting the calming sensation to course through your body. Your thoughts drift away. You don't try to follow or catch them. With each breath you take, you are feeling more and more serene. Breathe in, welcoming peace and harmony to your soul. Breathe out, exhaling all the negative energy and releasing your control. Realize how good it feels to be so relaxed.

Focus on being as relaxed as you can be at this moment. Allow your mind to settle down a little, too quiet, to be still. Instead, focus more on your body. How does it feel lying in your bed? Examine the coziness you feel beneath your sheets. Feel how smooth your sheets are and the gentle weight of your blanket on top of you. Relax in the embrace of the softest bed in the world. You are content in every way.

Imagine that on the other side of the room is an open fire crackling. The orange and yellow flames emanate a sensation of calmness as its soft light can be seen upon your walls and ceiling. You feel the warmth of this sensation. You watch closely as the flames flicker and dance upon the logs. The sound of the crackling fire reminds you that you are safe in this space. In this bed you are warm, cozy, and protected.

Scan your body for tension. Find where you still hold stress in your body. Examine your shoulders, your neck, your temples, and your back. Find the stress that is hiding and release it. Allow your body to feel relieved, relaxed, at peace.

Examine the aroma of the fire as it fills the room. The fragrance is deep and musky. It reminds you of good memories with the ones who love you. These memories remind you that your life is beautiful. Place both hands on your stomach, one below your ribs and one above your belly button. Take a deep breath in through your nose, inhale those good memories. Let the air fill your belly and your hands rise on top of your abdomen. Then, through your nose, exhale all of the negativity you have collected. The worries that you harbor are no longer welcome here.

Breathe in the relaxing scent of the fireplace; fill up your stomach like it is a balloon. Let your hands move as you inhale. Then exhale any remaining tension. You now feel loose and at ease. There is a calmness that envelopes your body as you breathe. As you feel more relaxed, you hear only the fire in this quiet space. The quietness of the room also quiets your mind and you welcome rest and relaxation.

As you lie down, keep breathing and reveling in this blissful setting: you're tucked inside your cozy bed with a fire to keep you warm. Focus on this serene moment and give yourself permission to enjoy it. Remember that you are in control. Many times, your mind is over thinking, overanalyzing, and too critical. In this moment, it is you who is in control, and you will exhale those negative thoughts. As you exhale, you regain your balance, and you feel content. Your body feels looser, lighter, and a weight is lifted off your chest.

Your body is light and warm as you listen to my voice. Let me guide you as you drift off. I'm going to count now, and you will listen. Let my voice lull you. You are safe and relaxed and warm.

Ten... Your body is entirely loose and relaxed.

 Nine... You are in a peaceful, calm, and safe environment.

Eight... You can feel the warmth and love of those who care about you, enveloping your senses.

Seven... The sound of the burning fire, the crackling of wood lulls you further into an even deeper state of relaxation.

Six... You inhale all of the good in the world with each breath you take.

Five... You exhale all the bad, expelling all of your stress and anxiety with each breath out.

Four... You feel your body getting lighter until you are almost like a feather in the breeze.

Three... You feel your mind becoming heavier and brimming with warmth and love.

Two... Accept the peace that has engulfed you, understand that it is good. Let it send you off ever deeper into the feeling of relaxation.

One ... You feel yourself drifting all the way down, as deep as you can go, nearer to the bottom, towards warmth and sleep.

You are safe and you are relaxed. Allow yourself to feel safe and relaxed in this space.

Instead of the ground, you see that there is a quiet pond below your tree and soon you will touch the surface. As you float towards it, you notice its stillness. There are no ripples or disturbances. The surface is smooth and clear; it is as reflective as a mirror. As you reach the water, you greet the surface with a delicate kiss.

You send gentle, peaceful ripples from your contact. Concentric circles echo out to the edges of the pond. This energy radiates from you until the last ripple falls away. It is now you on the water, undisturbed and immersed in the tranquility of your setting. You drift on the surface of your unconsciousness. You feel the warmth of the water beneath you and surrounding you. The water is so soothing that you feel yourself getting heavier. You feel as though you could keep floating deeper and deeper beneath the surface until you fell asleep.

SLEEP HYPNOSIS SESSION 2

Bubbles

Begin by taking a breath in and shifting your body into a relaxed and comfortable position. Close your eyes. Let your hands be open by your sides with the palms facing up. Your legs slightly apart. Breathe in through your nose and breathe out slowly. Turn your head to the right, and then to the left. Now, back to the center. Breathe in and breathe out. Feel your belly rise and fall with your breath. Throughout this meditation practice, if your mind decides to wander, notice the distraction and return to my voice. All you need to do right now is allow yourself this time to de-stress and let go of all the tension that you feel in your body. Let go of all worries, thoughts, and emotions. Let yourself relax and become one with this moment. Nothing else matters. There is no right or wrong way to proceed, so follow along and let your body do as it will as naturally as possible.

Now, state your Sankalpa. Think about what is genuine, positive, and present in your life currently. For example, "I can tackle anything that comes my way." Along with your breath, repeat your intention three times.

Breathe in, "I can tackle anything that comes my way," breathe out. Inhale, "I can tackle anything that comes my way," exhale.

In, "I can tackle anything that comes my way," and out.

Bring awareness to your body. Remain completely still and notice the sensations that you feel as we go through each body part. You might feel tingly sensations. You can also feel stressed or tense muscles. You can even feel restlessness or relaxed muscles. Whatever you might be feeling, just become aware of it and move on to the next body part without much thought.

Let's begin with the face. Visualize your facial muscles and the tension you hold in your face. Become aware of your forehead, ears, eyes, scalp, and temples. Bring awareness to your nose and nostrils. Your lips, cheeks, and chin. Your jaw, teeth, tongue, and throat. The back of your neck. Breath in and breathe out.

Now, become aware of all the sensations you can feel in your upper and lower back. Your buttocks, the backside of your thighs and calves. Notice every part of your body that is in contact with the floor. Now, become aware of your ankles, feet, and toes. Pay attention to any sensations or tension you might feel in your chest and abdomen. Follow your belly rising and falling with every breath. Now, your shoulders and arms. Your left shoulder, arm, wrist, palms and fingers of your left hand. Now your right shoulder, arm, wrist, palms and fingers. Imagine there is a light caressing your body. Follow this light to the tops of your thighs. Follow it right down to your feet and toes. Sit here a moment, taking in each breath and each sensation. You are very self-aware at this moment. Do not judge or label any sensations, just notice them.

Now, bring your attention to your breath. As you inhale, notice the air travels through your nostrils, into your lungs, and into the depths of your stomach. As you exhale, notice the out-breath. Notice how it ventures out of you, either quickly or slowly, yet naturally. It's like a wave. As you breathe in, this wave takes everything in. As you breathe out, the tide carries all tension away from you. You are feeling relaxed. Inhale. Notice all the sensations you experienced earlier. Exhale. Notice all these sensations escaping from your body. Breathe in relaxation. Breathe out all your stress. Breathe in serenity. Breathe out frustration. Breathe in a positive light. Breathe out negative worries and fears. All you have is now. All that matters is right now.

Now, remind yourself of a time when you felt most panicked. Feel every symptom of losing control. Your heart is racing. Your world is spinning. Your breath is quick. Your body is tense. Sit with this moment without judgment. Do not label it as good or bad. Feel the tingling sensations of panic rush through your body. Look at this panic and fear from a third-person perspective. Watch as the anxiety runs its course. Take a deep breath in. Exhale slowly.

Now, imagine the fear and hostility inside you disappears. It is replaced with calmness and tranquility. It's as if the flick of a switch turned the alarm off. Notice that your body feels calmer and lighter as you breathe in relaxation and peace. Let all the fear and control wash right over you. You are now fully incapable of feeling fear and panic. Instead, you feel loosened and pleasant. A positive shining light starts flickering from the middle of your stomach. Imagine this light warming your center and expanding outward. It fills your whole body. Now it brightens the room around you. This light gets bigger and warmer until it engulfs your whole house. Breathe in, and as you breathe out, capture this relaxing warm light back into the very center of your core. You are at peace now.

Remember the feeling of this warm, positive shining light within you, and know that you can revisit it any time you want.

You are in an open field where there is no one around but you. There are no mountains, no hills, no trees, and no rocks. All that surrounds you is green grass and flat open lands where you can see for miles and miles in all directions. You feel the air surrounding you is warm and comfortable. You look down and see in your hand that you are holding a bottle full of bubble solution and a bubble wand. You take the bubble wand and dip it into your bottle of bubble solution. Then, you hold the bubble wand up to your mouth and blow. Out comes a neon pink, elephant-shaped bubble. It starts out small but gets much larger as it floats out from your bubble wand. You do this again, only this time, out comes a lemon-yellow, cheetah-shaped bubble. Watch as the cheetah chases the elephant. You blow another bubble.

This time, it comes out as a multi-colored rainbow bubble. The rainbow bubble becomes so big it forms directly above you and shines in the sunlight. You watch as the elephant now chases the cheetah. You blow another bubble, and an electric blue bumblebee flies out of your bubble wand. You watch as the bee circles the rainbow and buzzes around the cheetah and elephant. You make another bubble. This time, a golden-brown, bright green, royal purple, and flaming orange dragon comes out. You keep blowing the dragon bubble. It becomes bigger and bigger. First, the wings, the body, the head, legs, and then the long-spiked tail. The dragon is so big that you feel a gust of wind almost blow you completely over when it flaps its wings. You reach out to touch the dragon. POP! Pop! Pop! All of the bubbles have popped.

Remember the statement you made at the beginning of this exercise? Now, state your Sankalpa again: "I can tackle anything that comes my way." Along with your breath, repeat this three times.

Breathe in, "I can tackle anything that comes my way," breathe out. Inhale, "I can tackle anything that comes my way," exhale.

In, "I can tackle anything that comes my way," and out.

Bring your back attention to yourself. Notice every part of your body that is in contact with the surface below you. Feel your body melt and relax back into this surface. This surface pushes back as it gently supports all of your weight. You will not fall. You are completely safe. Breath in and breathe out. Bring your attention to the room you are in.

Is it a bedroom? A living room? Breath in and breathe out. Visualize your ears. What do you hear? Pay attention to all of the sounds around you, both near and far. Notice the sensation of the air against your skin. Wiggle your toes and then wiggle your fingers. Now, move your eyes behind your eyelids without opening them. Breathe in. Breathe out. Open your eyes and look around the room. Take a moment before you sit up or move too much. Become aware of this very moment.

FOLLOW YOUR PATH - SESSION

Gently close your eyes and allow your body to lie flat on the floor. Breathe in slowly. Breathe out. Notice your surroundings. What can you hear? What can you smell? Notice how you feel. What can you taste? Pay attention to your surroundings; what you can hear, smell, feel, and taste. Listen to your thoughts. Do not judge them. Just become aware of them. Feel your emotions one by one. Breathe in slowly. Breathe out and let go. Let go of all that you are holding within yourself right now. Breathe in slowly. Breathe out and let go of all that negativity. This moment is yours. This time is yours. You deserve to feel peace. You deserve to feel pleasure. Make sure that you are completely comfortable. Move your head gently from side to side and then, back to center. Focus on the feeling of your breath. Breathe in through your nose and breathe out. Notice your belly rise and fall with each breath. Rise and fall.

Think of something that your heart desires and that you wholeheartedly believe in with your entire being. Think of a statement or intention for this exercise. For example, "I am bold and brave." Repeat these three times with everything that you believe. Feel this with every part of you.

Breathe in. "I am bold and brave." Breathe out. Breathe in. "I am bold and brave." Breathe out. Breathe in. "I am bold and brave." Breathe out.

Now, bring your focus to your left toes and foot. Notice whatever sensations might be there. Now focus on your right toes and foot. Notice the feelings happening here. Visualize your entire right leg. Following from your foot to your leg, notice anything that you might be feeling in your right leg. Ankle, calf, shin, knee, thigh, right buttock, right hip, and hip bone. Now, going from your left foot and toes, follow any sensations you might be experiencing up your left leg. Ankle, calf, shin, knee, thigh, left buttock, left hip, and hip bone.

Bring your awareness to your center, above your pelvis, and below your chest. Watch your belly rise and fall with your breath. Make sure you are breathing as naturally as you can. Do not take deeper breaths than you need to. How does your lower back feel? Your upper back, back of the neck, chest, front of the neck? Notice anything you may be experiencing without judgment, and do not label any sensations as good or bad. Notice them and move on. Bring attention to your left shoulder. Your upper arm, lower arm, wrist, palm, fingers. Visualize what your palm and fingers look like. How are they connected? Now bring your attention to your right shoulder. Your upper arm, lower arm, wrist, right hand, and finally, your fingers and thumb. Let go of any tension you might be feeling right now.

Move on to the bottom of your face. Relax your jaw and unclench your teeth so that they are not touching. Notice the sensations in your lips as you breathe in and out of your nose. Become aware of your nostrils and nose to the middle space between your eyes. Your eyelids, temples, left ear, right ear, forehead. Relax all the muscles in your face so that you hold no expression. Breathe in calm air. Breathe out all of the tension you might be feeling.

Inhale for a count of five. One, two, three, four, five. Hold for three seconds, two, three. Exhale all of the air at a slow and steady pace. Two, three, four, five, six, seven. Continue breathing out, and when you are finished, breathe in again. Repeat these two more times.

Don't be alarmed if your mind wanders. Notice this and bring your attention back to your breathing. Become curious about the breath you are taking. Where is it coming from? How long does it last? What does it feel like? Slowly, return your breathing back to an average pace that feels natural to you. Notice all of your tension is released from your body. Inhale and allow yourself to be at this moment. Exhale and let go of everything that is worrying you right now. Nothing else matters. Just breathe in and out naturally.

Now, imagine you are outside in a blistery snowstorm. Feel the cold breeze brush against your skin in waves of gusting winds. As you breathe in, feel your lungs become cold as ice as if you were sucking on an ice cube. As you breathe out, visualize the icy breath that escapes your cold lips. Take this moment in with your entire body.

Feel your bones and lungs ache from the fresh, frosty air. Be here in this moment right now.

Now, imagine you have walked inside with a comforting fire ready to warm your soul. You are instantly hot. You are sitting in front of a fireplace now. You hear the wood snapping. You smell the fire bake the kindling. You taste the warmth in your throat and on your tongue. You feel the warmth radiating from the flames. You are so warm that it's as if cold never existed.

Be here in this moment right now. Inhale and exhale slowly and at a comfortable pace.

Imagine that you're walking down a nature trail. All around you, bushes, trees, flowers, and animals come to life. Animals are following you and chattering in their animal squeaks. Trees are welcoming you further with every step forward. In the distance, you can hear a stream of water as if it is guiding you to move forward. The sunlight is peaking at you from the canopy above, and the ground feels sturdy and inviting. You see a deer twenty steps ahead of you, it has stopped in the middle of your path. Bunnies, squirrels, raccoons, lizards, and smaller rodents are on either side of you, leading you forward. As you come closer to this deer, she takes a step toward a little cottage right in front of you. The door opens as you come close.

You step inside this cottage, and directly in front of you is a staircase. This staircase swirls up as if it goes on forever. You hear the door quietly shut behind you, as all of the sights and sounds of nature disappear. You are in complete darkness. You take a deep breath in and focus your vision on a light two steps in front of you. You take one step up, another, then another. All you can see is the bluish-white tinge of a light guiding your way. You reach out to the wall to your right and grasp the railing to your left. The staircase starts to bend around. All you can see now is the next step ahead of you. As you come closer to the top, this light starts shining brighter and brighter. Soon you are almost at the top, and the light becomes so bright that you need to hold your arm in front of your face. At the very top of this staircase, you reach a door. Before entering, you inhale deeply and exhale slowly.

You open the door and step through. You are now on a cloud. The sun is so bright, it's hard to see. The wind embraces your skin, and the warmth leaves you motionless and peaceful. This cloud takes you away from the door in the middle of the sky and lower to the ground.

As you come closer to the earth, you see houses and people as small as ants. You see lakes, mountains, forests, and cities all beneath you. A few minutes more and the cloud brings you to the ground at your house. You step inside your home, and the cleanliness of your favorite scent fills your nose.

Remember the intention you made at the beginning of this exercise. We are going to repeat it now three times.

Breathe in. "I am bold and brave." Breathe out. Breathe in. "I am bold and brave." Breathe out. Breathe in. "I am bold and brave." Breathe out.

Visualize yourself walking to where you are now from your front door. Notice the walls, the hallway, your roommates, children, or spouse. Notice where they are. Walk into the place where you are right now and see yourself lying down again. Feel the surface you are lying on. Feel every place in your body that is in contact with that surface. Feel it supporting you. You feel safe. B1-ing your attention to your ears. What do you hear? Follow the sound, notice which room these sounds are coming from. Bring your awareness to your breath now. Where is it coming from? Is it warm or cold? Is it slow or fast? Breathe in and breathe out. Become aware of your fingertips on either hand. Wiggle them. Become aware of your feet. Wiggle your toes. Let your legs roll in and out gently. Slowly roll your whole body to your right side. and back to the center. Now, roll your whole body to your left side. Now, return to lying on your back. Bring your head upward, so your chin is tilted up. Now downward, so your chin is touching your chest. and then, back to the center. Now turn your head to the right. Then to the left, and now, back to the center. Bring your attention to your face. Then lie regularly and open your eyes.

HYPNOSIS FOR DEEP SLEEP SESSION

Welcome to a deep sleep session. I am going to assume that you are lying in the comfort of your own bed or someone else's bed. Please cover yourself up with a comfortable duvet if you are cold or lay on top of the duvet if you are getting hot. Fluff your pillow before we begin because I want you to start in the most comfortable position possible.

Switch the light off and become aware of the background music in this session. Isn't it soothing? Allow your thoughts to flow with the calm rhythm of the sound you hear. As you fade the sound of the music just slightly, you grab onto the sound of my voice. Listen to the sound of my voice and the background music in harmonious balance. I want you to close your eyes. Your eyes are feeling droopy now. You have had a long day and your eyes are allowed to feel heavy. Keep your eyes closed and use your sense of hearing to follow my suggestions. You feel a deepening trust in my instructions with every word I speak. Allow my suggestions to flow through your mind, bringing more comfort with each moment.

You are going to focus on your breathing now. I want gentle inhales and exhales. Keep a consistent rhythm with each breath you take. Feel your body soften further with each exhale. Stop thinking about the thing that just crossed your mind and come back to me. I want you to feel a small wave of guilt for allowing your mind to wander. Now start breathing over again. Small, shallow breaths-gently in and gently out. Keep doing this till you maintain an even rhythm. Allow your breathing to slow your heartbeat, one breath at a time. Your eyes are feeling more and more drowsy with each beat of your heart. However, something is keeping your mind from giving into your fatigue. Your mind refuses to shut down and you don't know why. Shift your focus back to your breathing now and follow the air as it flows into your body. You can feel your body rise and fall as you inhale and follow the flow of air as it exits your body. You are becoming more confident in this session.

I want you to focus on your surroundings once your breathing is even and relaxed. What do you see? You only see darkness, but this darkness seems to beckon you. There is a strange comfort in it. I want you to focus harder this time. Listen to your body inhaling and exhaling as you lay there. Indeed, there is something appearing in the darkness. What is it? It's just a little white speck.

Now I want you to focus on your body. Think about the way your head feels. Does it feel heavy? Strain your muscles a little and hold them for a moment. Feel the tension release from your muscles as you slowly relax them. Now your head feels clearer and more comfortable. Do the same with your neck. Make your muscles tense in your neck and hold for a moment. Count to three in your mind and then you may release them. Can you feel the tension of the day dissipate? All the horrible stress leaving your neck area. You feel more relaxed now.

Bring your focus back to the darkness for a moment before we continue. What do you see now? Oh, the white speck looks like a light, a very distant light. Can you hear any sounds yet? No? I didn't think so.

Shift your focus back to your body and pay attention to your arms this time. I want you to make tight fists with your hands and hold them. Now you can count to three again before you unclench your fists slowly. Allow yourself to become aware of the sensation of your action. Focus on the negative energy that is leaving your hands. Your arms feel relaxed now.

Go back to the darkness now. What do you see? The light has come closer now. Oh, but wait, you can hear a distant sound now too. I want you to focus on that sound for a moment. You feel excited to find out what the sound is but with much focus, you still can't identify the sound.

Okay, come back to me again. I want you to pay attention to your stomach muscles now. Pull your stomach muscles and hold them for a moment. Keep holding them. Count to five this time and release. Focus on the comfort and relaxation the release has brought you. You are reaching a level of comfort that is strange to you. Welcome this newfound comfort.

Please go back to the darkness. I need you to know that I am here with you every moment of this session. Don't be afraid of anything. What do you see? The light has drawn nearer again. It's bright now and you can't quite make out what it is. Hear my voice speak calmness over you as the light approaches. The sound is getting louder now too but it's a disturbing sound. It would normally make you worry. However, you are not worried right now. You feel a deep-seated sense of safety in this session. Even though this feels strange and familiar at the same time, you know you must have been here before. You are finding it easier to overpower the sound with the calming background music now. Keep your focus on the music and the sound of my voice.

Let's return to your body once more. I want you to shift your attention to your legs. If you are not too far into your relaxation, I want you to move your ankles from side to side for a moment. Count to three and stop. Now you may pull your muscles stiff. Please don't strain them enough to injure yourself. Hold them like that for three seconds before releasing them. Pay close attention to how soft your legs feel now. You are in a deep state of relaxation, a state of mindfulness.

Now I want you to focus on your breathing again. Make sure it remains steady. Feel your body conform to each inhale and exhale. Your arms are too relaxed, and you don't feel the need to touch your body to feel this. You are in an unfamiliar state of mind now. You have become one with your subconscious mind. You feel a deeper need to trust the sound of my voice now as the time draws nearer. All doubts have swiftly removed themselves. It's just you and my voice now.

Follow me back to the darkness that you have been curious about. There is a certain level of calm in this darkness. As it comes back into your inner sight, you see exactly what the light is. As a matter of fact, the sound is clear and distinct now. You are blinded by the light heading straight at you and deafened by the screeching noise. My voice is never silenced by this unbearable noise coming closer to you. The sound of metal grinding against metal makes you shift your attention to where you are standing. The bright light shows you the tracks beneath your feet. Your mind wanders off to an old western movie you've seen where someone looked like a deer stuck in headlights. Please bring your concentration back now. You feel your heart skip a beat for just a split second when suddenly, a great sense of calmness comes over you. You feel safe and accepting of this huge metal train coming your way. You are fully capable of stopping it dead in its tracks.

This train is filled with memories that plague your sleep every night. It's also filled with worries about tomorrow, the stresses of today and various other thoughts and feelings. This is your own speeding train of thoughts that disrupts your sleep every night. A monstrous metal machine that won't leave you alone. This train comes to take away your peaceful darkness every night after you reach the first stage of sleep. It's a menace that makes you sit up for hours, fighting your heavy eyelids. The sound of this train alone is enough to drive anyone mad. It's the first time you are facing it directly, identifying it, visualizing it.

Now I want you to concentrate hard on the background music and the sound of my voice. Keep your breathing steady and use welcome sounds to drown the noise out. You know you can do it. Breathe in gently and breathe out slowly, one breath at a time. Listen to the calm tone of my voice and allow it to reassure your comfort and safety. Nothing will happen to you because you are stronger than you think. You know that this train is nothing more than a figment of your imagination. You also know that all those worries in the cargo can be dealt with tomorrow. There is no need to face this train now. Tomorrow is another day and trains shouldn't be running this late. You know your thoughts will be clearer when tomorrow comes.

Now listen closely to my suggestion. Allow every word to resonate through your mind. You have created this train; you have brought the image to life. Only you have the power to erase this image. Your imagination has brought it to life and your imagination will remove it. Now take your attention back to your breathing and focus on your heartbeat. Can you feel the steady rhythm of every beat? Take a moment and count your beats. Follow each beat and feel how it pumps the calmness through your veins. Now I know you are ready.

You stand on the train tracks, facing the oncoming train and know that you are now in control. You can control the trains' every movement. You make the train slow down as you watch the sparks on the tracks from the train's brakes. The sound doesn't even penetrate your hearing anymore because you have drowned the sound out now. You can feel the vibrations in the tracks as the train draws nearer but you have no fear. You cannot fear something that doesn't exist in a physical form. You dig deep into your subconscious and find the strength you need to make this train vanish.

Suddenly, you are transported back into complete darkness. A darkness that feels safe and peaceful. You have successfully stopped the train and you're alone now. No thoughts or worries can cross your path anymore. Your physical form is feeling feather light now. You are connected to it and don't need to leave your darkness anymore. You feel proud of yourself, and you have never felt this tired before. Your mind is still connected with your subconscious mind. Give your subconscious mind permission to leave you now. You will be perfectly fine in this quiet space. There are no more possible disruptions. You can feel yourself floating into a deeper, more peaceful state of sleep (Sealey, n.d).

SOUNDS OF NATURE SESSION

It is going to be a nice night tonight. Before you fall asleep, I will take you to the most beautiful beach you have ever seen. This place will relax you and calm you down to your very soul.

First, take a nice deep breath, getting into a very comfortable position. Rest your head upon your soft pillow and take another deep breath... relaxing in bed, loosening all muscles.

Breathing deeply, letting your legs relax and sink into the bed... breathe fully, letting your torso melt into the mattress... breathing, completely let go the muscles in your neck and shoulders, letting you head be cradled by the pillow... take one last deep and relaxing breath, as you exhale let your eyes gently close.

Good...

Relax your body even more by letting go of any areas of tension... breathe in again slowly... release the air with a whooshing sound, like a wave crashing on the sand...

Become more and more relaxed with each breath...

Breathe in again very slowly... pause for a moment....and let it go...

Feel your body giving up all tension... becoming fully relaxed... enjoying every moment of this calm and peaceful breathing...

There is a gentle wave of relaxation flowing through your body... down and up... up and down... just like the waves of the great ocean...

It flows from the tips of your toes, through your feet, up your ankles and lower legs... through the knees, thighs, hips and pelvis... relaxation flows through your abdomen, chest, back and shoulders ... down each arm, relaxing any tension... all the way down to the hands and each fingertip... it flows up your neck, relaxing you entirely... the back of your head fully relaxes, your facial muscles let go completely... and the very top of your head, including your brain, becomes deeply relaxed...

Breathe in slowly and deeply again... releasing the air with a whooshing sound... and as you do bring into your mind the thought of a white sand beach.

The sand is warm... and as soft as velvet under your feet...

The waves of the turquoise ocean in front of you are making a gentle whooshing sound, just like your breath...

This beach is surrounded by tropical forest. You can hear the song of beautiful birds being carried through the air... you notice the leaves on the palm trees are moving with the wind, making a soothing rustling sound... you can hear crickets and tropical frogs enjoying their life in the rainforest.

Notice the different greens of nature, the beauty in the way that each leaf reflects the sunlight.

You can feel the gentle warmth of the sun on your skin, relaxing you. This place is the definition of tranquility. The ocean water is shallow from a distance; then far out along the horizon you can see the water gets a rich, sapphire blue.

There are white fluffy clouds in the sky that resemble the blossom of cotton in its raw form...drifting by, slowly in the sky. The sun's rays alternate between warming your skin and being hidden behind the passing clouds.

The beach sand turns into giant rocks to your left, which soar into tall caves along the water's edge. As you walk towards these caves, you feel the sand moving under each footstep... you gaze behind you and see a long strand of your footprints trailing behind you. The rock formations get more massive as you draw closer ... as you draw near the cave, you find yourself under the shadow of its cliff, and the air becomes cool from the shade.

There is a large opening in the rocks... it is a welcoming entrance.

As you go inside the cave, you can hear the ocean waves become amplified as they bounce off the rock walls. This cave is magnificent. You can hear trickling water, so you follow it to find its source. Along the interior wall of the cave, fresh water is springing from rocks, making the most relaxing sound of moving water you have ever heard. This water seems to glow, although there is no sunlight reflecting in the cave, it shimmers with light before your eyes.

You cup your hands together and gather some of this water, bringing it to your lips for a drink. It is the purest and most refreshing water you have ever tasted. It nourishes and replenishes you... hydrating every part of your being with its beauty.

The tropical birds know of this water source, and make their way flying into the cave, chirping their beautiful song. There are all different types of birds, large and small. They land on the floor of the cave and drink the fresh water that is collected in various puddles below. Bringing their beaks down, scooping the water, then raising their heads high to allow the water to trickle down their throats. They are not afraid of you; it is almost as if you are part of their flock.

These magnificent birds are co close, you can clearly see the beautiful rainbow of colors that make up their feathers ... bright reds... yellows... greens... and turquoise blues that match the water of the ocean. Their eyes are surrounded by the crisp white of their skin, and they look directing at you with kindness and curiosity. After getting their fill of hydrating water, they fly out of the cave and back into the rainforest.

You take a moment to sit down in this cave, there is the perfect shape rock protruding from the ground that almost resembles a bench. Have a seat and close your eyes for a moment, tuning into the sounds around you....

The waves... the distant birds... the tricking fresh water... the breeze... each sound soothes you to your very soul. Take a deep breath in and hear the air going in and out of your lungs... you can smell the clean saltwater...

(pause)

Open your eyes and see the cave towering above you... what a beautiful spot.

You are ready to go back out and explore the beach, because it has gotten a little cool for you here...

As you make your way out of the cave, the cool rock under your feet turns back into sand... you pass into the sunlight and feel the sunrays begin to nourish your skin. The water is so clear and inviting that you decide to go for a little swim. The sand becomes firmer under your feet because it is saturated with sea water... waves come closer and catch your feet. At first, the water seems cool, but actually it is the perfect temperature. The waves rush up to your ankles, and your feet are being buried in the sand as your weight presses you down into the earth.

You make your way into the water and can see that it is shallow for a long distance. It goes to just above your waist. Curious to see what is going on below the surface, you decide to dip your head under the water. As you do, you find that allowing yourself to become weightless in the ocean is one of the most serene experiences in your life.

Without hesitation, you open your eyes underwater to find that you can see perfectly clearly, without any discomfort.

In front of you, there is an immaculate reef, teeming with fish. You swim closer, finding that you do not have an urgency to go up for air. It is almost as if you are a tropical fish in this ocean.

As you swim closer to this city of underwater life, you see that the colors are more brilliant than anything on land. It is almost as if you are witnessing the rainbow manifesting as life. Everything you see is alive... moving in the ocean's gentle current...

Small, yellow fish with black stripes notice your arrival... they look at you with curiosity in their eyes, and excitement in their swimming. Then they travel back down into a giant pink sea anemone... you can see that this is their home. Several yellow fish pop in and out of the living home, dancing about... it is almost as if they are showing off their home.

A large purple fish with bright glowing green spots catches your eye... swimming slowly by with confidence and grace. They notice you, but do not seem to be phased by your appearance...

You are witnessing every color you can possibly imagine in your view of this reef... from the blackness of the pupils of the swimming creatures, to the shimmering white light of the sun cascading through the water like a diamond prism.

Everything is peaceful here at the shallow reef.

You are ready to head back to the shore to enjoy a walk through the sand when you suddenly see a mighty sea turtle approaching close by... the way its arms and legs push it through the water makes the turtle weightless, though you know he could easily weigh more than you. The sweetness in its eyes comforts you down to your soul...

Just when you thought this experience could not get any better, you see there is a trail of baby turtles following behind. You think by the size of this sea turtle, it was a male, but now you can see the gentleness that could only be embodied by a caring mother. Her hatchlings have made the daunting journey into the expansive ocean. They are vibrant and ready to take on life. This is only the beginning of a long lifetime along the reef.

You are grateful for this experience in the reef, and it is time to head back to the beach. Getting out of the water is effortless because the waves are gentle, and the water is shallow.

The sun begins drying your skin.... the clouds are passing by ever so slowly... you are beginning to feel tired from taking in all the beauty around you, and it just so happens that a plush beach recliner is positioned facing the water, with a large white umbrella providing just the right amount of shade...

You have a seat and position yourself on the chair so that your muscles can let go... you are fully ready to take a long nap in this paradise. Inhale the sweetness of the air... exhale into complete tranquility... hear the nature behind you.... the ocean in front of you... and the breeze all around you...

You see the cave you were exploring earlier in the distance and can remember the crisp taste of the fresh spring water...

You can feel the cushioned beach chair supporting you... Every part of your body and mind are at peace, and deeply relaxed...

Gazing out upon the big blue sea, you notice the horizon, and how it is the only perfectly straight line in the landscape... You enjoy the precision of how the ocean meets the sky.

Take in a few more deep breaths as you lazily keep your eyes open, enjoying the sights of this beach paradise.

Breathing in deeply... relaxing more and more... exhaling into serenity...

Breathing in fully... let your body sink down, melting any last bit of tension away... exhale into tranquility...

Continue breathing slowly... Allowing the breath to lull you into a deep sleep... slowing down more and more....

Allow my voice to fade into the distance now as you drift off to sleep... Goodnight...

COUNTDOWN TO SLEEP SCRIPT

Begin by preparing yourself and space. When you are ready, lie down in your bed, flat on your back - adjusting pillows and blankets as needed. Place your arms at your sides with your palms facing downwards.

Once you are comfortable, gently close your eyes.

Focus all of your awareness on your breath. Just notice what it is doing? How does it feel? Where is it flowing?

What sensations do you experience in your breath?

As you focus in on these sensations, let yourself begin to slow down your breathing. Allow each inhale and exhale to lengthen and deepen, using your abdomen to guide you into a relaxation response. Feeling your stomach rise on the inhale and fall on the exhale. If you notice you are breathing in more through your chest than your abdomen, take this time now to adjust this. Breathing in through your belly triggers a sense of calm, breathing in through your chest triggers feelings of increased energy. If you notice yourself breathing in through your chest, intentionally make the switch to feel the air rising and falling more from your stomach than anywhere else in your body.

You have control over your sense of peace in any given moment. As you breathe in slowly and deeply, be proud of yourself for being here - for doing this work. You are strong. You are powerful. A person tapped into their ability to relax and sleep deeply is naturally powerful. This is an incredible strength.

Take a deep inhale in through your abdomen and begin to feel a sense of deep appreciation towards yourself. Hold your breath at the top, and when you are ready, exhale with a long audible sigh. Feel gratitude for your ability to work on improving your sleep. Feel appreciation towards yourself for all that you are in this moment. Appreciating your breath, your brain, your 5 senses: the abilities to taste, touch, smell, see, and hear Feeling appreciation also for your physical and emotional abilities, your interests and your hobbies, your skills, and your talents, who you are as a person. There's so much about you that is worthy of appreciation.

Breathe into that and let your mind continue to identify that with what you appreciate about yourself.

Let yourself use your exhales to relax even further and more deeply into this moment. With every exhale let go of tension in your body, and with every inhale welcome in a thought about your day that causes you to have feelings of gratitude. This could be the tiniest thing, from getting a green light in traffic, to going to the coffee shop and having a delicious cup of coffee, to having a table to eat off of, a bed to lie in, or simply finding a lucky penny on the floor. You could even feel grateful to have air to breathe.

It doesn't matter how big or small, in this moment take your time to feel gratitude towards everything in your life today that has been going well. Let yourself think of everything from the moment you woke up, all the way to this moment now. What is there to appreciate?

What good things happened today? And what good things happened to those around you?

With each inhale think about all that you appreciate today, and on each exhale, let yourself sink more deeply into a peaceful, sleepy feeling.

Let your heart swell with appreciation as you continue to reflect on every tiny little thing that went well today, as you realize your life has so much goodness in it.

Now think about the people in your life who bring you gratitude. Who are they?

What have they done for you?

See their faces and feel your love and appreciation.

With every exhale let yourself sink into this feeling more. Notice yourself letting go of any and all tension as feelings of gratitude overcome you.

It's like you're counting sheep but instead counting all that you have to appreciate in your life.

Each person or situation coming to mind brings more peace and relaxation to your heart, body, mind and soul.

With gratitude overflowing from your heart, notice the heaviness of your body in this moment.

Feeling the weight of yourself lying down. Feeling as though your eyes are glued shut and your body is anchored down to the bed.

As you feel your body entering into very deep peace, you notice your mind becoming loose and perhaps less focused. It's okay if the words you are hearing come and go from your awareness as you begin to drift off.

Let yourself listen only as long as you can, allowing your body and mind to fall asleep as they are ready.

With your body completely relaxed, your breath slow, your heart full of gratitude, you begin to countdown your favorite moments in life, bringing yourself into more and more peaceful deep sleep as you count. We will start from 10 and work down to 1. As we reach number one, you will be completely asleep and at peace. Each number brings you more and more relaxation.

Ten.

See a person from your childhood who brought you great joy. Who are they? What do they look like? How do you feel in their presence? Let yourself recall the scenes and the feelings of being with them.

Notice yourself relaxing into this imagery and emotional state. Letting your exhales bring you deeper into the peace of this memory, as we countdown to nine.

Feel yourself relaxing even further as you see a place you used to love to visit as a child.

Walk: around in this space, noticing the colors, the shapes, the smells and the sounds. As this place becomes more vivid to you, you relax even more, feeling the goodness of this memory washing over you.

Countdown now to eight.

Sinking more deeply into this moment, recall a memory that brings great joy, from any moment in your life. Breathe into how you felt at that time in your life and let yourself embody that feeling. Let that joy fill you entirely and you relax even more heavily into the moment.

Counting down again...

Seven. Begin to feel appreciation for something you accomplished in your youth. Something you are proud of. Something that brings you joy to think of. What did you do? Why does this make you feel good?

Feel the peace and relaxation of letting yourself drift off into this pleasant memory, as you relax even further while we countdown to six.

Notice your body growing even heavier, as you let yourself feel into the feelings of the beliefs that you hold most dear in life - of what you stand for, of what sets your heart into feelings of passion. Let the goodness of connecting with your passions swell within you, just letting yourself feel this way without thinking too hard about it. Just letting the feeling envelope, you, as you embody it while your physical sensations grow heavier, more relaxed.

As we countdown to five...

Let yourself feel the feelings of who you most want to be. The feelings of how you want to feel every single day. Let peace envelope you. You know who you are, and the feelings you most desire to experience in this lifetime, as you relax in this moment. These feelings envelope you as you sink into them...and we countdown to four.

Noticing your body, even heavier, and yet now also somewhat lighter. Feeling as though it is drifting away, drifting into the most peaceful sense of relaxation. And as your mind drifts, and you reflect on all of your skills and strengths and interests, and who they serve you in this lifetime, you take these feelings while you relax even more as we countdown to three...

You let your free-floating mind answer the question: who am I really?

And as you drift off, you let the answer fill your body. Not in words, but in emotions and in a physical sensation of love and peace. And that love and peace wraps you up, as you countdown to two...

You are practically asleep now, if not already, as you answer the question: why am I here?

Let the answer fill your bones. Again, not in the form of words, but in the form of emotions. And as those emotions fill you, you feel yourself drifting off as we countdown to one...

And in this moment, you fall asleep, feeling the most profound appreciation for all that you are.

HYPNOSIS FOR A MORE ENERGIZED MORNING

Hypnosis helps you to find success because it can retrain your brain to think positively. It is natural to see the negative aspects of life. There's nothing wrong with that, and you should not feel guilty over involving thinking negatively about a situation. We all do this as humans.

These hypnosis sessions won't be the answer to getting the negativity out of your life. They will help to awaken your senses and realize the positivity that exists all around you. By consistently practicing hypnosis, you will discover that you can find the good within the bad, always looking on the "bright side" of things.

Positive Thinking Hypnosis

I want you to take your right hand and make a fist. Nothing too tight, nothing too loose. Lift your thumb and your pinkie out from the rest of your fingers, holding this hand gesture while you start to become aware of your breathing.

Take this hand now and place your right pinkie over your left nostril. Press your nose so that you can no longer breathe out of this nostril. Breathe in through your right nostril now.

Then take your right thumb and place this on your right nostril, releasing your pinkie from the other one. Now, breathe out through your left nostril. This is going to help keep you focused on breathing. Repeat this several times until you feel more relaxed. The more that you do this, the more relaxed you will feel.

As you breathe in, envision that you are breathing in positive vibes and breathing out all of the bad. Everything that you feel cycles through you just like air. The negative vibes will always fade away.

From this moment forward, each breath of fresh air will be a new positive one that you bring into your body. Each breath out will be one that helps you to let go of every regret and other negative perspectives that you are holding on to. You continue to breathe in good energy and breathe out the bad.

Each thought you have, you will now find a way to turn into a positive one. Even neutral thoughts are ones that can breed positivity. This isn't going to warp your perspective negatively. You don't have to worry about having an unrealistic perspective. You will always have an idea of what reality looks like.

You will be focused on finding the positive even in situations that seem to present the biggest challenges to you.

Each positive thought that you have is one that helps you grow an even stronger mindset. Always remember that the more that you grow positively, the more positive outcomes that will come your way. You are focused on seeing the good in everything.

You recognize that there are two sides to every story. You will not only see one side. However, you will see that the positive side is the one that is beneficial to your overall perspective.

You continue to focus on your breathing, realizing that this is helping you to relax. The more relaxed you feel, the easier it is to be positive. You are letting go of all the tension that is being held within your shoulders. You are releasing the tension that you carry on your back throughout the day.

You start to see how even stress can be a positive thing. Stress is something that helps you to put an emphasis on the things that are the most important in your life. Stress is something that isn't fun to experience. However, knowing what it feels like helps you to enjoy the moments that you are relaxed even more. Though stress can be difficult to feel, it is a reminder when you are in a good mood of the negative feelings that you don't have to experience within that present moment.

With each breath you take, you become more and more relaxed. The calmer you are, the easier it is for you to see the positive in everything that surrounds you. As negative thoughts come into your mind, you are able to turn them around easily.

When something comes into your head that fits in with a negative perspective, you look at the way in which you can change this pattern of thinking. You are not concerned with keeping up a toxic outlook on life. There is nothing beneficial that having a negative perspective has helped you with so far in this life.

You are letting go of negative emotions. You are moving forward away from the things that have happened in your past life, and you are not letting this become something that will affect how you view your future.

Though certain things that you have experienced have caused you to question your outlook and this great world, you are highly aware that there is so much positive that you have not seen simply being there.

Think of something in your past that has happened that was challenging to deal with at that time. What is it that might have been something in which you wish you had changed?

How can you twist this thing that you might feel regret, guilt, or remorse over and turn it into a positive thing that has helped you to grow to be the person that you are now?

If you can take a past experience and turn it positive, then you can be confident knowing that no matter what might be coming your way in the future, you will always know how to twist it positively and use it to your advantage.

You recognize that many of the negative thoughts that come into your head aren't even your own. Many of the negative perspectives, harsh judgments, and toxic assumptions that you might make or have made in the past were ideas planted in your brain by those around you. You might have had toxic relationships, negative people, or unhappy individuals in your life that have created the judgments first. You might also be someone who has struggled with the many negative perspectives in our society.

You are not concerned with keeping up with these negative ideas anymore. They don't do anything except provide more anxiety to the perspective you have now that you are working so hard on building in a positive light.

You continue to become more and more relaxed, assured, and calm with your positive perspective.

By being able to twist even your most negative thoughts into something positive and useful, you have discovered that it becomes that much easier to have a clearer perspective overall. You are not blinded by the fear and anxiety that can sometimes come along with having a negative perspective.

The only thing that you are focused on is finding the truth. From there, you can twist it into something positive that will help you grow. The things that are harder to remember or live through are all things that played a huge role in the development of your character.

You are allowing positivity in your life because it is something that will consistently help you to move forward. When you are thinking positively, then more positive things will come your way. It will become much easier to achieve the things that you want.

You are going to keep up with hypnosis because you know that it will be something that will continually aid in a new perspective and a healthier outlook on life overall.

You feel your entire body relaxed now, but it is your mind that is the most at peace. The more relaxed you are, the more positive thinking you will allow in your mind. The more you exude positivity, the less you feel anxious.

You feel good knowing that it is OK to be positive. You will still see the negative side sometimes, and you will not be blind to the truth. You will be focused on taking what you can from a situation and using the most from it, helping you even further to remember what needs to be focused on the most.

You feel good about yourself, and you feel good about the world. You are hopeful for the future and no longer let one small instance define your overall perspective on even larger ideas. You feel powerful, you feel assured, and you feel prepared.

Continue to focus on your breathing as you slowly come out of this hypnosis. Remember the "thumb and pinkie" trick on the days that you might be feeling like you need it the most. Keep track of your breathing now as we count down from twenty. When we reach one, you will either be out of the hypnosis or ready to move onto others and potentially even sleep.

Finding Abundance Hypnosis

This hypnotic exercise is one where I really want you to focus on the abundance that you are going to find within your lifetime. To start, let's make sure that our breathing is in perfect rhythm. Find a comfortable position and don't allow any distraction in the room in which we will be conducting this hypnosis.

We are going to be breathing in "threes." What this means is that I am going to count to three repeatedly. Each time I change, you will switch from breathing in and breathing out. Keep your hand in front of your mouth for the fast few. This will be so that you can feel the air that comes out of your body.

Breathe in for one, two, and three. Breathe out for one, two, and three. Again, breathe in for one, two, three, and out for one, two, three.

In, one, two, three.

Out, one, two, and three.

In, one, two, three.

Out, one, two, and three.

You can place your hand down. Continue this breathing in for one, two, three, and out for one, two, three. In, one, two, three. Out, one, two, and three.

The point of feeling your breath is for a physical reminder of your strength and your power. Without even putting effort into it, you are continuing to keep your breathing rhythm each and every day.

Now, let us move on to visualization. Picture your dream home. Whatever it might look like, imagine that you are standing right in front of it. Maybe it is in a penthouse in the heart of New York. Perhaps you prefer a cabin in the middle of nowhere.

Now step toward this dream home. Walk up the stairs and into the front door. As you open the door, you discover that it is filled with the most amazing decorations that you could ever have imagined. The living room has a large TV that you can watch your favorite movies and shows on. You move into the dining room and see a massive table that is big enough to hold every last one of your friends.

You move into the kitchen, where you see pantries and cupboards filled with goodies, snacks, and other types of foods that you can have whenever you want. The floor is clean and smooth beneath your feet. The walls are clean and have pictures of those you love and who love you. You have unique art that no one else does, and everything about this home reminds you of the abundance that is present in your life.

CHAPTER 4

Meditation Explained

MEDITATION AND THE MIND

Meditation, being a personal practice, has many different ways through which it can be exercised. The most common types are focused attention or the mindful meditation whereby one focuses on a specific thing such as how to breathe, the body sensation or even an object that is far or next to you. The whole idea behind this kind of meditation is to help one focus strongly and specifically on one point and to try to have their attention back on this one thing when it wanders.

Open monitoring meditation is another form of meditation that is often used, whereby one pays attention to everything that is happening around you. This helps one to notice everything without necessarily having to react. This type of meditation helps one to fit well in a work environment where the colleagues might be the type that overlook things. It equally aids mothers with small babies to pay attention to their children. Children tend to want to be everywhere doing everything. If a mother is a type that reacts to everything they notice, then they may end up being depressed, confused and always worried.

A friend, I will call her Jane (not her real name) opens up and explains to me how her dad would always convince her to meditate. This began way back when she was only 15 years of age. She always felt this meditation idea was so vague and just not her cup of tea. With lots of persistence from her dad, Jane decided to try out this whole meditation thing and find out what fancy it carries, but by this time she was an adult already.

Jane made up her mind, but she said she was not going to give it her all and to her, two minutes per day were just enough, yes, "two minutes!".

Jane had read somewhere that when you start something, start it off as a tinny habit and that is what will make it consistent hence achievable. She knew so well two minutes were too few to make much difference, but at the same time, she felt that was the right place to start from. After some time, Jane was able to realize that it may not be easy and simple but had enormous benefits to her day-to-day happiness, and this new habit transformed her mind completely. Jane says that it is good that many people feel proper meditation should last at least 15-20 minutes, but meditation is not a test of how strong one is; instead, it should focus on developing a long-lasting habit. Two minutes is simple, and one can grow from that by increasing the time gradually.

What happens to the brain when you meditate?

Scientists agree that meditation is the number one brain changer in the world because it is the neuroscientific most proven way, which can upgrade the human brain. Meditation nurtures the brain. We have read that meditation is a critical pillar in mental health, because it lowers stress levels and reduces the levels of anxiety. From previous studies done, meditation and mindfulness bring forth positive physiological changes which link reflection and the brain more profoundly.

As time goes by, meditation is becoming more conventional. Many people are starting to appreciate the art of spending time working with their minds. They are learning to follow their breath and understand the power of the now moment. Meditation is currently being practiced in many different places like schools, homes, workplaces with various groups coming up, while others are at an individual level.

Different brain regions are enhanced through meditation, and here are some of them:

Parietal lobe - It is the part of the brain that controls how one feels; it is highly connected to emotions and loneliness. It is well understood that any healthy human being needs to sleep well, eat right, and do exercise in order to be in good shape and be happy. We are connected through relationships within a family and outside the family. Every human being is a social being in need of mental, emotional, physical balance and well-being. Science speculates that when one feels connected with the people around them, it strengthens immunity by lowering the levels of anxiety and depression while raising the levels of self-esteem and empathy. The average human mind has a tendency to focus on the past and worry about what tomorrow holds, without just focusing on the present and what the present has to offer. Having too much time alone can have practical mental and physical health consequences.

Meditation trains one to overcome this lonely feeling by allowing them to focus specifically on the magical moments. The magical moments are those specific moments when one is with one's beloved family playing games, sharing jokes, eating and drinking, those moments when you are lost from your problems, and you do not care about tomorrow or the next five minutes. Those moments that you can pay anything to have back, and you will not regret the amount of money you spend. Friends and family may not always be present with you, but meditation is one thing that will always be at your disposal. The human brain is divided into two hemispheres whereby every hemisphere has its right to perceiving, thinking, remembering, reasoning, willing, rejecting, and emoting. Scientists say that the people with the left side brain personality tend to be more logical, practical, and analytical and are better in science and mathematics-related subjects. The right-side brain personality people are very imaginative, intuitive, and sensual with high excelling power for philosophy and arts. However, neurologists confirm that those people who are highly creative in many things that they do, use the whole brain and not just the right or the left side. These types of people tend to be very successful and massively creative because they use both halves of the brain in an integrated and balanced way.

With meditation, it is possible to balance the brain and yield many benefits to an individual. Through meditation, the neuro cold war is terminated, leading to brain hyper-connectivity, which in return integrates the left and the right sides of the brain hemisphere. When the brain hemispheres are harmonized, benefits such as improved focus, super thoughts, creativity, excellent mental health, enhanced memory and concentration, and clearer thinking in all issues.

Other effects of meditation are as explained through the following concepts.

Hippocampus "Happy."

It is at such times that we say meditation brings an end to depression. There are several people who suffer from major depression related complications. In fact, research suggests that out of fifteen people, one person is depressed. With numbers increasing, many people are up in arms to find the cure for depression. The more someone gets depressed, the more the hippocampi shrink. It is similar to when one breaks a leg then the size and strength of that leg slowly wastes away inside our orthopedic cast. The first step to lift oneself out of depression is to try and ensure the hippocampus has strengthened and is not wasting away. Here is where meditation comes in handy because it is the certified hippocampus personal trainer. In one specific study, the findings revealed that after eight weeks of consistent meditation, the left and right hippocampi of the people who were taking part in the study had a significant growth percentage of the neural thickness, density, and overall size. With such findings it is evident that one can add meditation to one's daily routines and be able to reverse the harmful effects of depression no matter how deeply rooted they might be. At the same time, it helps to prevent any further damage that may be caused by depression since the hippocampus is equally the brain memory center.

Hippocampus "Remember Everything."

The hippocampus is responsible for the skills that improve memory and learning abilities even through old age. Many of at times we have found ourselves in situations where we have forgotten where we put our keys, what a friend's name is, and a birthday for a close family member, and in some cases, we even set passwords and forget a few days later. Old age causes memory loss among people. A prominent neuroscientist has done several studies on the meditating brain. He found that meditation has the ability to dramatically and drastically increase the hippocampal cortical thickness. To make it clearer, just the way an artist would mold clay, meditation is one of the things that shape the learning and memory center of our brains into what we can say is a beautiful thing. Even though our intelligence to some extent is set the day we are born, meditation has enhanced one's ability to remember everything to the level that everyone would very quickly say you're an intelligent person.

Anterior Insula "Compassionate"

Nothing is satisfying and makes one happy like when you can be compassionate or kind to someone. People believe that what makes us truly happy is when we are achieving and receiving a good and great thing, but that is not true. According to research, true happiness comes from the actual practice of compassion. When we get the opportunity to help someone, and we do it, we get the right feeling of being connected to the world. That moment when we offer without having expectations of receiving anything in return, we feel happy and satisfied from the act. It is evident from when a mother holds her child for the very first time, she does not expect to receive anything in return, but still gets a unique satisfaction in giving life to life. It is for the same reason that mothers are never tired of whatever they do; they do it to the best of their ability with or without the support of their husbands. No wonder it is said that a mother is a true reflection of real love. Spreading joy throughout the world may not be enough but practicing compassion and kindness is what opens doors to a bulk of health benefits like lifting depression, alleviating anxiety and strengthening immunity.

New day places before us a golden opportunity to spread and share love. The spread of kindness is more comfortable said than done, but meditation is what launches our compassion consciousness into an orbit of love. Being compassionate and kind may never put a Nobel Prize on your shelf or table, but one thing we are sure it will do is that it will undoubtedly put a smile on the other person. If this is spread to others, then the world will be a better place to live in. The little things in life are what make the world a better place like the butterfly effect. Always putting yourself in other people's shoes and seeing yourself through other people's eyes can spark a tremendous positive change in people's lives, into the family, into the community and this will spread to the world.

MAIN TECHNIQUES FOR MEDITATION

You can start by visualizing a beautiful calming and serene atmosphere or environment. You can also move to a deserted place that is free from any element of destruction. These techniques achieve the best results if they are done at night. Meditation for sleep helps you start preparing for rest and puts any stress behind you. Anyone who can keep their anxiety levels low during the day usually experiences better sleep at night.

The following are four of our fundamental techniques of meditation for better sleep.

Abdominal Breathing

This involves regular breathing exercises at intervals. While breathing through the abdomen, you need to pay attention to your breath, as this will help you relax both during the day and at night. Well, some people practice abdominal breathing in a poorly lit room with low ventilation while others prefer a bright room with open windows. Look for things that calm you down and clear your mind like soft music. You can put on headphones as you listen to music. As you lie in bed, put your hands on your belly and notice its movements as you breathe in and out. Watching the progress of your hands on your stomach helps to calm you down from all the evil thoughts of destruction in your mind. Breathing exercises and relaxing songs can help calm anxious people. This is because they are at a level of anxiety that, if not controlled, can cause adverse effects. Focus your hands on your abdomen and you can also hold your breath then release it gently. As you do this, notice the abdominal and hand movements when you release your breath. Do this continuously until the specific time that you set for the end of the meditation.

Guided Imagery

For some people, the imagination of accomplices can help them offset the meditation exercises. There is no specific rule on what you should imagine. Your creativity should be based on something that calms you and relaxes your body. The following are some of the things that other people find calming: clouds, mountains, and oceans. Identify a place where you feel safe to use your imagination and invite all the senses to help you explore. The brain does not usually understand the difference between reality and pretense. For instance, if you start imagining lovely food, it is possible to begin salivating. Another scenario is watching a scary movie that can make you imagine being part of the film and experience whatever the actors were experiencing. Guided imagery can be accomplished alone or through the help of a specialist. Some of the specialists may include behavioral therapists, hypnotherapists, cognitive therapists, and sleep doctors. The therapist can help with imagination as you listen to their voice, telling you where to go.

Mindful Meditation

There are so many aspects of your life you should focus on to achieve mindful meditation. During mindful meditation, you let your thoughts go and focus on one thing at a time. Understand that it is essential to let go. If you can write a journal every day with all the issues that are disturbing your mind, you will reduce your anxiety level. Writing these down during the day also helps you deal with your problems early, so that you do not carry some of these thoughts during meditation at night. Mindful meditation mostly concentrates on how the brain processes things and coordinates with the mind. It has been used not just for anxiety alone but also as a remedy for depression and eating disorders. Mindful meditation helps focus on breathing, which then brings the attention of the mind to the present without having to drift into concerns of the past and the future. By doing this, it helps one train their daily thoughts to come up with relaxing responses. You can set around 15 minutes for meditation during the day. This, in turn, creates a reflex that will quickly form a great sense of feeling relaxed. This will then trigger a relaxation response during the night when you find it hard to sleep.

Counting Down

As you continue lying in bed, fix your gaze upwards. Looking up, one can strain their eyes, and that strain can relax you. Counting down can begin from counting the belly breaths. After this, proceed to a moment of progressive calmness and relaxation. You can then move down the staircase before going to your peaceful quiet space.

Going to bed at night with many thoughts regarding worrying over a particular problem may rob you of a peaceful night of sleep. Millions of Americans are affected by regular disturbance during sleep caused by having difficulty falling asleep. This, in turn, makes them very sleepy during the day. When one is tired during the day, their productivity can be low, and it can harm their health if it is not controlled. Meditation for sleep helps incorporate simple exercises that allow the mind to relax and the body to calm down, thus making one fall asleep faster and easier.

Tips for Falling Asleep During Meditation

Before you start meditation for rest, ensure that you are getting peace before you begin sleeping. Comfort can mean perfect meditation styles, proper postures, and better breathing exercises.

The following are some of the tips that can help one fall asleep during meditation for deep sleep:

Be Consistent

It is essential to be consistent in meditation for deep sleep since your body and mind will need constant changing and reassurance that all will be fine. Taking your time every day to practice meditation trains your mind and body that you will have to sit down or lay down and be still.

Cool Down

After a long rough, anxious day, we all want to jump in our cozy beds, snuggle under the blankets and sheets. The foundation of a happy frame of mind and good health lies in getting good quality sleep.

Consider calming focus, like the sound of your breath, a positive sound or phrase, or a prayer. If you are more interested in sounds, say them louder repeatedly daily as you inhale and exhale. Do not be distracted or worried about whether you are doing okay. If your mind wanders away, take a deep breath as you slowly bring your attention to whatever you chose to focus on.

Manage Your Anxiety

Meditation for sleep is not just merely for falling asleep faster, but it also helps deal with issues related to anxiety. Stress interferes with sleep and sleeping patterns of an individual. As you experience irregular sleeping patterns, so does your body struggle to stay awake during the meditation process. Determine your stressors and come up with ways of managing your anxiety without letting it interfere with your meditation process. Managing anxiety means you will have to reduce stress and deal with things that stress you the right way. When you can put your anxiety under contra you will be able to improve the quantity and quality of your sleep. Better and more sleep will make you feel well-rested and wake up very re- energized to face the day.

Meditation is the first recommended remedy to reduce anxiety and its effects. Other things can also help mitigate anxiety, like good exercise, moving out of harmful relationships, clearing debts, and changing careers.

Identify the source of your stress which in turn causes your anxiety and deal with it. Managing anxiety will help improve your sleeping pattern, and in turn, make you have a better-quality lifestyle.

Have A Specific Bedtime Routine

The best thing about the method is that it keeps you grounded, and it imprints some structures and regular patterns in the brain. Consistency is also crucial because it communicates with the body at the right time to wake up, and when the body feels drowsy and wants to sleep. People who work in shifts often find it very difficult to have a consistent bedtime routine. The more anxious a person is, the harder it will be for that person to fall asleep. This is because the mind is not at rest since it is disturbed and unsettled. All anxiety patients should understand that there is some level of anxiety that they may have no control over. Instead of blaming yourself for always feeling anxious, forgive yourself, and be positive about meditations. By doing this, you will have already started the healing process without knowing. If it helps, you can keep a journal and write down your stressors, how they made you feel, and how you handled them. Meditation for sleep, therefore, ensures that when one goes to bed, their mind is free and ready to relax.

BENEFITS OF MEDITATION,

HOW MEDITATION CAN HELP YOU

Building Self-Awareness

For starters let's focus on self-awareness.

Take a minute and honestly ask yourself how aware you are of how your body reacts to specific situations. How do you react to light? How do you react to fear? How do you react to happy events? Take a minute and identify each of these physical manifestations of your mind and evaluate them - why do you react in this way? Have you always acted in a specific manner? What has changed, if anything?

You may notice that as you go through these questions in your mind, other questions and thoughts will enter your mind that you didn't anticipate. This is actually very typical and natural. Often times even if you think that a specific thought or specific trigger will cause your mind to think or work in a specific manner, in reality, it doesn't necessarily process the information in any specific way. This is why reverse psychology works on certain individuals and backfires on others - not all people react to the same form of stimulus in the exact same manner. Meditation allows you to practice introspection and truly identify how your mind reacts to specific triggers. It's almost as if your mind is doing a mental inventory of how you think, how you process, and most importantly how you react.

Try to think of meditation as a form of mental yoga - here the objective is to forge a stronger link between the mind and body. This is to ensure that your mind is more aware of how your body is responding specifically to cues. Meditation helps us understand our own individual sense of awareness. Helping ground us in the present moment allows us to act and think in a way that keeps us in the present.

Reducing Stress and Anxiety

This is just one benefit -meditation is not intended to enhance one's sense of self simply. In fact, a major reason why so many people get involved in meditation is because they wish to use the practice to cure themselves of unwanted stress and anxiety that they might be dealing with.

Let's simplify this, shall we?

Why do you think you are invested in meditation?

What do you feel unsure or nervous about starting your meditation program?

Try answering this instead - in the past week what are five negative things that have impacted the way you act, think and react? Make a shortlist in a separate journal. Have you listed them for yourself? Good! Now ask yourself how often one of these thoughts has controlled your mind. Let's say you feel unhappy at work - how often have you thought of quitting? A lot?

How often do you think about how badly you want to change jobs? Almost always?

Most importantly how often have you done something that would help you change your job, or extract yourself from that toxic work environment? Odds are you just said never very quietly under your breath. Whether or not you feel like you are ready to admit your thoughts to other people, you yourself know exactly how often you are sometimes even obsessing over the negatives in your life. Do you ever wonder why you don't feel comfortable telling other people how often these negative thoughts come to your mind?

Think about it - if you don't like admitting how you are thinking, odds are that you already know, subconsciously or at some level, that what you are doing isn't good for you. Always keep in mind that while negative things will continue to happen in your life, how far you allow that negativity to spread into your personal space is a decision that you are making constantly. There is always a more productive way to deal with negative thoughts - if you feel you are stuck in a bad job, instead of obsessing over the negative features of the job entails, train your mind to focus on the way out. Line up for new job interviews, consider talking to the human resources department or a supervisor; the point here is to actually actively do something instead of just letting things happen to you.

Taking control of the negativity that surrounds you is a key part of ensuring that you lead a healthier and happier life, because this negativity is what breeds stress and causes anxiety to build in your mind. So, if you really want to live a stress-free, healthier and most importantly, happier life you are going to want to start by finding a way to reduce your stress levels, and train your mind to focus on productive activities, instead of the anxiety triggers that you have built for yourself.

Honing Mental Clarity

Another common issue many individuals tend to have to deal with is - the lack of clarity that is predominant in today's world. For the most part, research has shown that multiple mental disciplines, such as yoga and meditation, can help control the mind and even improve it. Conditions such as ADHD, which is a form of attention deficiency, have been known to show significant improvement with meditation and meditation-based activities.

While it is common knowledge that physical exercise can help keep the body in shape, what people tend to forget is that the brain needs the exact same thing. Neuro exercises or mental training activities can potentially keep our brain in shape, and can also weed out certain undesirable mental characteristics, such as depressive thoughts, or anxiety.

One of the fundamental issues currently being studied by scientists is the subject of neuroplasticity. What is neuroplasticity, you may ask? Well, simply put, scientists have begun to discover that, contrary to popular opinion, an individual's brain is not shaped at the time of their birth - in contrast, the brain is actually constantly growing and learning, which is why it is possible actually to change our brains to specific forms of mental training. For example, one can retrain the brain to alter or improve multiple personality quirks, such as how attentive you are, how happy you are, how angry you are etc.

Instead of considering emotions such as happiness, anger, or disappointment individual reactions, think of them as skills. You can train your mind so that you are more skilled at being happy or positive, although odds are you have subconsciously been training your mind to be the exact opposite. Neuroscientist Richard Davison, of the University of Wisconsin, conducted a three-month research program on the impacts of the Vipassana form of Buddhist meditation that deals with increasing mental clarity, and improving sensory awareness. On completion, he found that volunteers who had received Vipassana meditation as a form of mental training, were much faster in their ability to identify and focus on detailed information. In contrast, individuals who had not participated in the training seemed less clear and less stable in their ability to retain information. Because of this, meditation is now being seen as a form of mental exercise that helps individuals take advantage of the plasticity of the human brain, in a quantifiable and scientific manner.

Building Focus and Fortitude

However, it is not just mental clarity that is affected by meditation. In fact, a large part of meditation deals with building focus. While the science of the issue has clearly established that meditation can help enhance mental clarity by playing with the neural plasticity of the mind, it also does so on a more chemical level by releasing specific hormones to help counter your stress levels.

When you are stressed out, your body releases certain hormones to let your mind know that it is overloaded. Once your mind starts to register that you are stressed out, the body then starts to release adrenaline because it thinks that your body now needs more energy to help get you through these backlogged tasks. The only problem here is that adrenaline can work against you. While theoretically adrenaline should be helping you to get better and to do your tasks quicker and better. Adrenaline serves an important function in our bodies, but unless we learn to control stress, adrenaline works against us. Instead of helping us get through stressful moments, excessive adrenaline instead increases anxiety, and multiplies our stress reaction.

Keep in mind the release of adrenaline in your body is a physical reaction to fear or danger, or some sort of immediate desperate need - this is a physical reaction, that has been passed on to us from our ancestors, who at the time needed that extra bit of energy to fend off predators or to stay alive. Now imagine having that level of pressure put on you every single day, because you are unable to distinguish between a life-and-death situation, and a workplace crisis. Your body simply doesn't know the difference.

This of course is where meditation steps in. Meditation gives us a sense of self-worth and power, so that when we are faced with a challenge, we are not immediately dropping the ball and going into "danger" mode - instead we are calmly teaching ourselves to cope, which in turn allows our brain to focus and develop better coping strategies.

Have you ever given yourself a social media detox? Is your immediate reaction after you wake up to check Facebook? One of the first things you might want to do is slowly detach from your phone or the distractions of social media over the next seven days.

Meditation teaches your brain to do the exact same thing in terms of the topics on which you are focusing. By slowly teaching yourself to focus on the factors which you would like, such as positive outcomes, you simultaneously build your mental fortitude. You're training your brain to not go into panic mode at the slightest thing. At the same time, you are also teaching yourself how to react to those smaller, yet persistent mental problems that you find yourself facing on a daily basis. Win-win!

Emotional Intelligence

So, what else does meditation help with? Well, for starters, it is also an extremely important tool in the development of emotional intelligence. As you begin to become more aware of your own self and how you react to specific situations, you will also realize that you are attuned to how people around you react to those same situations. This form of awareness is also commonly known as emotional intelligence and is currently considered to be of extremely high value. Indeed, some scientists have begun to prefer the evaluation of emotional intelligence over the evaluation of one intelligence quotient to determine a person's potential.

While you probably ask yourselves multiple times whether or not you are good enough or smart enough, odds are you probably don't ask yourself if you are compassionate enough or if you are a good listener. If you are familiar with the television program, The Big Bang Theory, you've probably seen that the protagonist Sheldon Cooper has been portrayed to be an individual with extremely high IQ, but extraordinarily low EQ factor. In later seasons, this impacts his career growth, as well as his personal life. This is actually extremely common - no matter how smart you are, in order to truly succeed in life, you will find that you will require a certain amount of emotional intelligence.

Mental Health Benefits

Unfortunately, there are many individuals who suffer from mental health issues. Whether you are dealing with anxiety, depression, or something along those lines; meditation can help place you in a better mindset when practiced on a regular basis.

Decrease Depression

In a study done in Belgium, four-hundred students were placed in an in-class mindfulness program to see if it could reduce their stress, anxiety, and depression. It was found that six months later, the students who practiced were less likely to develop depression-like symptoms. It was found that mindfulness meditation could potentially be just as effective as an antidepressant drug!

In another study, women who were going through a high-risk pregnancy were asked to participate in a mindfulness yoga exercise for ten weeks. After the time passed, it was found there was a significant reduction in the symptoms often caused by depression. On top of the benefit of less depression, the mothers also showed signs of having a more intense bond with their child while it was still in the womb.

Reduce Anxiety and Depression

In general, meditation may be best known for the mental health benefits of reducing the symptoms associated with anxiety and depression. It was found that through meditation, individuals who practiced meditation such as Vipassana or "Open Monitoring Meditation," were able to reduce the grey-matter density in their brains. This grey matter is related to stress and anxiety. When individuals practice meditation, it helps create an environment where they can live moment to moment rather than getting stuck in one situation.

While practicing meditation, the positive mindset may be able to help regulate anxiety and mood disorders that are associated with panic disorders. There was one article published in the American Journal of Psychiatry based around twenty-two different patients who had panic or anxiety disorders. After three months of relaxation and meditation, twenty of the twenty-two were able to reduce the effects of their panic and anxiety.

Performance Benefits

When you are able to relax, you are amazed at how much better your brain will be able to function. By letting go of stress, you leave room for positive thoughts in your head and will be able to make better decisions for yourself. It's a win-win situation when you can improve your mood and your performance simply from meditation.

Better Decision Making

A study done at UCLA found that individuals who practiced meditation for a long time had a larger amount of gyrification in the brain.

This is the "folding" along the cortex, which is directly related to processing information faster. Compared to individuals who do not practice meditation, it was found that meditators were able to form memories easier, make quicker decisions, and could process information at a higher rate overall.

Improve Focus and Attention

Another study performed at the University of California suggested that through meditation, subjects are able to increase their focus on tasks, especially ones that are boring and repetitive. It was found that even after only twenty minutes of meditation practice, individuals are able to increase their cognitive skills ten times better compared to those who do not practice mindfulness.

Along the same lines, it's believed that meditation may be able to help manage those who have ADHD, or attention deficit hyperactivity disorder. There was a study performed on fifty adults who had ADHD. The group was placed through mindfulness-based cognitive therapy to see how it would affect their ADHD. In the end, it was found that these individuals were able to act with awareness while reducing both their impulsivity and hyperactivity. Overall, they were able to improve their inattention.

Relieve Pain

It has been said that it's possible that meditation could potentially relieve pain better when compared to morphine. This may be possible due to the fact that pain is subjective. There was a study done on thirteen Zen masters compared to thirteen non-practitioners. These individuals were exposed to painful heat whilst having their brain activity watched. The Zen masters reported less pain, and the neurological output reported less pain as well. This goes to show that pain truly is a mental aspect.

Along the same lines, mindfulness training could also help patients who have been diagnosed with Fibromyalgia. In one study, there were eleven patients who went through eight weeks of training for mindfulness. At the end of the study, the overall health of these individuals improved and reported more good days than bad.

Avoid Multitasking Too Often

While multitasking can seem like a good skill to have at some points, it's also an excellent way to become overwhelmed and stressed out. Unfortunately, multitasking can be very dangerous to your productivity.

When you ask your brain to switch gears between activities, this often can produce distractions from your work being done. A study was performed on students at the University of Arizona and the University of Washington. These people were placed through eight weeks of mindfulness meditation. During this time, the students had to perform a stressful test demonstrating multitasking before and after the training. It was shown that those who practiced meditation were able to increase their memory and lower their stress while multitasking.

Physical Benefits

While mental improvements are fantastic benefits of meditation, physical benefits can help motivate individuals to begin meditation as well. Unfortunately, the standard of health is to turn to medication. If you are an individual who hates popping pills for every issue you have, meditation may be just what you need to help improve your health.

Reduce Risk of Stroke and Heart Disease

It has been found that heart disease is one of the top killers in the world compared to other illnesses. Through meditation, it's possible you could lower your risk of both heart disease and stroke. There was a study done in 2012 for a group of two hundred high-risk people. These individuals were asked to take a class on health, exercise, or take a class on meditation. Over the next five years, it was found that the individuals who chose meditation were able to reduce their risk of death, stroke, and heart attacks by almost half!

Reduce High Blood Pressure

In a clinical study based around meditation, it was also found that certain Zen meditations such as Zazen, has the ability to lower both stress and high blood pressures. It's believed that relaxation response techniques could lower blood pressure levels after three short months of practicing.

Through meditation, individuals had less need for medication for their blood pressure! This could potentially be due to the fact that when we relax, it helps open your blood vessels through the formation of nitric oxide.

Live a Longer Life

When you get rid of stress in your life, you may be amazed at how much more energetic and healthier you feel. While the research hasn't been drawn to a conclusion yet, there are some studies that suggest meditation could have an effect on the telomere length in our cells. Telomeres are in charge of how our cells age. When there is less cognitive stress, it helps maintain telomere and other hormonal factors.

Relationship Benefits

There are some people who are looking for a little bit more peace in your life. In the world we live in today, times can be very trying. There are constant deadlines, bills to pay, people to deal with; but now is the time to look at stressors in your life under a different life. Through meditation, you can become a more caring and empathetic individual to create a more peaceful life for yourself.

Improve Positive Relationships and Empathy

When we undergo stressful situations with obnoxious people, it can be very trying to remain empathetic. There is a Buddhist tradition of practicing loving-kindness meditation that may be able to help foster a sense of care toward all living things. Through meditation, you'll be able to boost the way you read facial expressions and gain the ability to empathize with others. When you have a loving attitude toward yourself and others, this helps develop a positive relationship with them and a sense of self-acceptance.

Decrease Feelings of Loneliness

There are many people who are not okay with being alone. Often times, we try to fill our time with activities so that we are never alone with ourselves. The truth is, it can be healthy to spend some time with yourself so that you can self-reflect on your life choices. In a study published in Brain, Behavior, and Immunity, it was proven that after thirty minutes of meditation per day, it was able to reduce individuals' sense of loneliness while reducing the risks of premature death, depression, and perhaps even Alzheimer's.

Along with feeling less lonely, meditation also opens up new doors to feeling a positive connection to yourself. When you love yourself, and you are happy with your own company, you may spend a lot less time on negative thoughts and feelings of self-doubt; both of which can lead to self-caused stress.

BREATHING FOR RELAXATION

Breathing for relaxation is a big part of guided meditation, and it's something that many people don't realize is a valuable skill for you to use in order to relax effectively. But, what's so special about breathing? How do you do it? Well, read on to find out.

Breathe!

You probably have been told when working to relax is to breathe or take a few breaths. This is often told when we're upset and worried. You might wonder why you should be told this when you're upset and worried, but it actually is beneficial when you're feeling anxious, and it can alter the speed of response to the body's breathing and anxiety. Diaphragmic is a breathing technique that is pretty helpful. It can create a developed feeling that actually communicates to our brain the element of safety.

I don't suggest using this immediately when you're super deep in an anxious moment, but you should, if there is a tough situation, use this in order to make a smarter choice when trying to figure out what to do next.

Plus, breathing is actually helpful for calming down, and it's a vital part of relaxing the body when you're trying to de-stress. Being able to breathe after a long day can be really cathartic, and it's something that lots of times people don't even realize they forget to do.

Breathing with meditation is essential, and there are a few ways for you to breathe effectively in a meditative sense, and luckily, we'll tell you how to do it here.

Diaphragmic Breathing

Also known as Eupnea or belly breathing is a breathing technique that helps to strengthen your diaphragm. Learning to Breath from your diaphragm is useful as it helps to relax the body, the breathing, and the like. Lots of times, we actually don't breathe from our diaphragm, resulting in shorter breaths that don't bring oxygen-rich air to the body. This results in people taking breaths that don't help calm down the body, and they aren't refreshing. Luckily, you can learn to breathe from your diaphragm, and we'll teach you how to here.

When you're using breathing for meditation using your diaphragm, you first and foremost want to sit with your feet planted on the floor or lay down. Put your hands right over your belly. From here, close your eyes, breathing in slowly and in a calm manner. Fill your belly with a normal breath, and don't breathe too heavily. You'll feel your hands move as you do breathe in like you're filling up a balloon. don't lift the shoulders as you inhale, but instead, work on breathing into the stomach.

At this point, breathe out to the count of five. Slow the rate of exhaling. After you finish exhaling, you hold this for a couple of seconds before you breathe this in again. Continue to work to continue the pace and slowness of the breath that is here. Do this for about 10 or so minutes, and practice this twice daily for 10 minutes each time. Do this routine regularly to help with your own personal meditation.

You can couple this with focusing on the breathing, and when an intrusive thought comes in, you can actually eliminate that thought by acknowledging it, and of course, letting it stick around till it's gone but not obsessing over it. But, if that's too hard for you, do take some time to just focus on learning how to breathe in an effective manner. It's something that's essential for learning how to breathe via your diaphragm and is important.

Now, a couple of points to take away from it are as follows. You should focus on your breath speed rather than the depth of the breath. don't catch your breath by taking in more profound ones, but instead, take it nice and slow.

Remember that with this, you won't be able just magically to turn off anxiety. That's not how this works, and instead, breathing will help you learn to relax and get through a tougher situation, and you can mostly use this as training to get into breathing in a calmer style with time.

Don't be afraid to practice this either. It takes a long time to master, but it does help immensely.

4-7-8 breathing

4-7-8 breathing technique is similar to breathing from your diaphragm but is kind of more of a timed step. It's good for people with anxiety and insomnia as it helps your mind and body to focus on your breath rather than thinking of your worries.

What you do to begin is you can either sit or lay down, and keep your hand on your belly, and then keep the other on the chest, similar to how you breathe from your diaphragm. But, what you do, is when you breathe in slowly, are you take in slow, deep breaths that go straight to the belly, and from there, silently count to four whenever you breathe in.

At this point, instead of exhaling immediately, you then silently count from 1 to the number 7. When you hit 7, you breathe out completely, and you count from 1 all the way to 8, getting all of the air out of your lungs. Try to get all the air out by the time you reach eight. At this point, you then repeat this once again until you feel completely calm. With this one, I do suggest you journal how you feel at the end of this, and also how you feel. Chances are, you're going to feel much calmer than you did beforehand. This is great especially if you're in a situation where you need to focus on the numbers, and if you tend to be the type that needs that to be grounded, I suggest using this.

Equal Breathing

Sama Vritti is similar to numbered breathing, proven to lower your stress and keep your calm as it balances out the mind. To begin, you breathe in for four counts and then breathe out through four counts. You should make sure that all of the breathing is done via the nose, and this is because it will build a natural resistance when you breathe.

This is basic pranayama, which is a type of meditative breathing, and this is used in many cases in yoga too. Some people like to increase their breathing by going to either six counts, or even to eight counts with the ultimate goal of calming down the nervous system, focusing more, and feeling the stress fall off your body. The best part about this is that it can work really well before bed, and if you feel anxious before you're about to sleep, this can be used to help eliminate distractive thoughts.

Alternate Nostril Breathing

Nadi Shodhana is a breathing technique that helps people with anxiety. This is an advanced breathing technique, great for relaxation as it clears your mind, calms your body and your emotions. This powerful technique allows you to balance out, calm, and also bring forth both sides of the brain. What you want to do is start in a sitting or lying down position, and take your right thumb, holding it over the right nostril. From there, breathe in, but also do it only through your left nostril. During peak inhalation, close off the left nostril with the ring finger at this point, and then, breathe out through the right side. This is a bit harder than you think, but it takes a little bit of coordination, and you can continue to do this by inhaling through the right and exhaling through the left.

This is a great one for when it's crunch time, and when you need to energize and focus. don't do this one before bed, because it won't really relax the body, but most will help get the energy away from the bad parts of the body and allows you to focus more. So, if you need to get yourself refreshed before you go through an anxious situation, this is an excellent one for you to try.

Skull Shining Breath

Also known as kapalbhati is an internal cleansing technique that can help rid of toxins in your body. It will detoxify, rejuvenate, and energize your body, but this is definitely one of the more complicated types of breathing. What you do is you start this off with an exhale that's super long, and slow as well, and then you follow this up with a powerful exhale that's generated. Once you get comfortable with the contraction, you want to inhale-exhale all through the nose for about 1-2 seconds for 10 seconds in total. This is the right one to wake up the body and shake off any negative energy. While it may not do you a lot of good in terms of overall relaxation, it's still a very vital type of breathing, just because it's an excellent way to relax the body from stressful thoughts, and it will allow you to have a much more conscious state, and in turn allow you to get a good feel for what you must do with your day. It's also good if you've got a lot of frustrations in your head, and you want just to clear them away. This is an advanced one, so I suggest not trying this until you're ready.

Roll Breathing

Roll breathing is another breathing technique that makes full use of your lungs as it allows you to focus on the breathing rhythm. You can do this in any position, but it's best to lie on your back with your knees bent upwards.

To begin, you can put the left hand on the belly, and then take the right hand, pushing it onto your chest. Take a moment to feel how your hands move when you breathe. What you want to do is fill up the lungs so that the belly hand goes up, and when you exhale, the chest hand is still. Breathe through your nose and then out through the mouth. Repeat this type of breathing 8-10 times. When you've done this enough, then add in the second step which is pretty simple. What you want to do is inhale first to the lower lungs area, but then, inhale towards the upper chest, breathing as slowly and regularly as possible. You'll notice that your left hand will fall as the belly falls, and the right will rise.

When you exhale in a slow manner through the mouth, you'll notice that you'll be making a quiet, almost whooshing sound as you first feel your left-hand move, and then the right-hand does the same. It makes you feel the tension leave the body, allowing you to feel more relaxed, and refreshed too. You want to do at this point is to continue to practice this for at least 3-5 minutes, and then notice that the belly and chest will rise and fall, almost like rolling waves, and you can also record how you feel. This is actually a great way to relax instantly.

As an aside, you may realize over time that you might be dizzy the first few times you try this.

STRESS AND SLEEP MEDITATION

Stress is a huge factor in whether or not you're going to get restful sleep, and it actually is probably the most major culprit when it comes to insomnia. This shouldn't be that surprising, but we'll go over why that is, and how sleep meditation will allow you to relax the body and reduce the instance of stress.

What Is Stress?

So, what in the world is stress? Stress is actually the "fight or flight" response when you're confronted with danger. Let's say that you're worried about an upcoming exam, or a work presentation. Maybe you start to feel a little bit apprehensive about this sort of thing, and you begin to worry a little bit. When you finally get it done, the stress tends to reduce, allowing you to feel better.

But we're often super busy and hit from all fronts with this feeling, this needs to either fight or flight, and this will make us feel anxious all the time. This stress starts to compound over time, and it certainly makes it harder for you to calm down.

Stress releases cortisol, which elevates the heart rate, makes the beta brain waves much more prevalent, and it makes your energy levels increase. It also releases adrenaline, which is a hormone that causes your energy to increase as well, but if you start to release this all the time, it actually can start to make you feel sleepy as well, and often, messed up adrenals are a huge part of a person's problems, and stress can cause a lot of issues with this.

So yes, stress isn't good for you if you're going to be stressed all the time. Now, if you're stressed once in a while and you use that stress to propel yourself forward isn't that bad, but if you're overworking the body in this front, it can cause a lot of problems for you in the future.

Stress and Insomnia

So how does stress cause insomnia? Well, stress is something that causes cortisol to be released. Again, it will elevate the heart rate, and it's the body's response to stress. This might be good if you need a little bit of an extra push, but when you're stressed all the time, this is how the body ends up staying up late, tossing and turning and not sleeping. Your body won't be relaxed, but instead on the edge all the time.

When you sleep, instead of thinking about the present, you're worried about the future. You're worried about how that presentation is going to go, your family, your partner, your life. You might end up feeling your brain go from one element to another, almost like it's jumping from one place to another. It's not good for you, and this then causes more stress so that more cortisol will be released, and more anxiety will start to form.

This is how insomnia is formed, and your brain just won't shut down. The best way to have a restful life is to have restful sleep and to help curb stress. It's important, since it actually can determine whether you're going to be going throughout the day dragging, or if you're going to be happy and restful.

If you want to sleep better, you need to curb stress. Now, it's nearly impossible just to make stress get up and walk away. Stress will be there, but there are ways to relax the body, and meditation is actually one of the best ways to help relax it, allowing you to feel better and to have a much better, happier life. You don't have to go through life constantly feeling stressed, especially when you're trying to sleep, so you should tap into what is making you stressed and start to work on relaxing the body so that you're not feeling this way all the time.

Meditation Helps

Meditation can do a whole lot of good on the stress in the body. It's actually a major means to help mitigate and in some cases, help to reverse the effects of stress. Stress is what causes insomnia, and meditation does a whole lot for the body in helpful ways.

How does it? Well, have you ever heard of the relaxation response? This is how the body responds to various factors that are used to relax the body, such as sedatives and the like. This is the complete opposite of the stress response, and if you're trying to help reduce the instances of stress when you're trying to sleep, it's a major part of it.

Now, the relaxation response is actually done by you. It's a volunteer response and your ability to help your body release the chemicals. You can have this become involuntary, but it's not that easy. However, if you do this, you'll start to relegalize everything is slowing down. That's essentially what you want to do. You want to slow everything down.

This actually will cause the blood flow to move to the brain, which in turn will allow you to improve the responses that the brain makes to different factors in the body. You know what else actually does this? Drugs. Sedatives that you take before you go in for a treatment or an operation do the same thing to the body that this relaxation does.

However, with those, you get side effects, and there are a few dangers to them, which is why I don't suggest fixing your sleep responses with drugs. However, meditation helps to relax the body naturally, and it also allows you to do this consciously. That's right, you're aware this entire time, and that makes a huge difference. You're the one who's deciding to do this, and it definitely can help you improve your sleep schedule and turn off the stress.

Guided meditations do a lot of good for a person, and guided sleep meditations will allow you to turn this on and turn the stressors off. Usually, with these you can feel the powerful effects that these have on your sleep, and it will gently lull you into a slumbering state. You'll notice with these that they have a little bit of vocals and music that allow you to relax and fall asleep. The tracks actually help turn the brainwaves that cause you to feel stressed and anxious. Instead, you'll feel restful, and one of the best parts of it, is you don't have to deal with this for a long period of time.

For just about 10 minutes or so, these guided meditations will help lull you to sleep in the way that you want it to. With this, you'll end up being able to turn the brain off in the ways that you don't want to think, and in turn, you'll feel happier, and much better as well.

Stress is something that we can't get away from. You often can't do that sort of thing, simply because it is hard to escape. Life isn't easy, and stress is a natural response, but if you're able to use sleep meditation in order to fix this, you'll realize that not only will you feel better, but you'll be less stressed, and much happier than you've been before.

TECHNIQUES TO TRY OUT

Starting meditation practice couldn't be less difficult. In its most essential structure, all you need is an agreeable seat, a cognizant personality, and to be alive. Pursue these means and become more acquainted with yourself better.

Locate a decent spot in your home or condo, in a perfect world where there isn't a lot of messiness, and you can locate some tranquil. Leave the lights on or sit in the normal light. You can even sit outside in the event that you like yet pick a spot with little interruption.

At the start, it sets a measure of time that is no joke "practice" for. Else, you may fixate on choosing when to stop. In case you're just starting, you can pick a brief span, for example, five or 10 minutes. In the long run, you can develop twice as long, at that point, perhaps as 45 minutes or 60 minutes. Use a kitchen clock or the clock on your telephone.

Numerous individuals do a session toward the beginning of the day and at night, or either. If you have the feeling your life is extremely occupied and you have a brief period, showing improvement over doing none. At the point when you get a little existence, you can do more.

Take a great stance in a seat or on some sort of pad on the floor. It could be a cover and a pad, even though there are numerous great pads accessible that will last you a lifetime of training. You may sit in a seat with your feet on the floor, freely leg over leg, in lotus pose, bowing - all are fine. Simply ensure you are steady and upright. On the off chance that the requirements of your body keep you from sitting upright, discover a position you can remain in for some time.

At the point when your stance is set up, feel your breath or some state "pursue" it - as it goes out and as it goes in. (A few variants of the training put more accentuation on the out-breath, and for the in-breath, you essentially leave a delay.) Inevitably, your consideration will leave the breath and meander to different places. At the point when you get around to seeing this - in no time flat, a moment, five minutes - return your thoughtfulness regarding the breath. Try not to pass judgment on yourself or fixate on the substance of the musings. Return, you leave, you return. That is training. It's frequently been said that it's straightforward; however, it's not that simple. The work is to continue doing it naturally. The results will accumulate.

Posture

Posture is the primary factor in meditation - regardless of whether we choose to meditate while strolling. The stance is regularly dismissed by apprentices and the individuals who meditate without an educator. A skilled contemplation instructor will never give the poor a chance to pose slides. Stance shields the body from encountering torment, from ill-advised arrangement, notwithstanding setting up the body for a meditative state.

- Take your SEAT. Anything that you're perched on - a seat, a contemplation pad, a recreation center seat - discover and detect that gives you a steady, strong seat; don't roost or wait.

- If on a pad on the floor, fold your LEGS easily before you. (If you as of now do some sort of situated yoga act, proceed.) If you are on a seat, it's great if the bottoms of your feet are contacting the floor.
- Straighten - don't harden - your UPPER BODY. The spine has a common shape. Give it a chance to be there. Your head and shoulders can serenely lay over your vertebrae.
- Place your upper arms parallel to your chest area. At that point, let your HANDS drop onto the highest points of your legs. With your upper arms at your sides, your hands will arrive in the correct spot. Excessively far forward will make you hunch. Too far back will make you firm. You're tuning the strings of your body - not very tight and not very free. What's more, it may not be as startling as you might suspect.
- Drop your jaw a little and let your GAZE fall delicately descending. You may allow you to eyelids lower. If you feel the need, you may cut down on them absolutely, yet it's not critical to close your eyes while ruminating. You can mostly let what appears before your eyes are there without focusing on it.
- Be there for a couple of seconds. SETTLE. Presently you can pursue the next breath that turns out. You've begun on the correct foot and hands and arms and everything else.

Customary meditation and Yoga stances have been created more than a large number of years, to consolidate legitimate breathing with the perfect arrangement of the vitality ways, inside the body. Put resources into a decent sitting pad, if sitting erect and straight, puts overabundance strain on the tailbone. Indeed, even the strictest of reflection experts may experience many sitting pads through an incredible span.

Patience

A significant advance toward appropriate reflection is to comprehend that contemplation requires persistence. It can take long stretches of committed everyday practice to arrive at the more profound degrees of awareness. A few people guarantee to have opened accessible routes to the more profound conditions of cognizance, yet these cases ought to be thought about while taking other factors into consideration.

Regardless of whether somebody built up an enchantment pill that could sling clients into the most profound thoughtful states, what great would it be? A significant portion of the reflective way is simply the adventure. Reflection requires some serious energy and practice. For specific individuals, it takes more time to clear the psyche than others. Much the same as Yoga don't compel it - simply make the most of your voyage.

Breath

Breathing must be done appropriately, and a factor that disrupts everything for some people is nasal blockage. The average individual can experience existence with their nasal sections swollen or blocked, and scarcely take note. In any case, a person who rehearses Yoga, or reflection, ought to be substantially more mindful of dissemination issues in their nasal locales. An extraordinary custom to perform, before contemplation, is nasal purifying. This should be possible, consistently, with a neti pot or sinus wash bottles, ensuring the nasal sections are clearly taken into account by breathing through the nose. It ought to be noticed that some nasal conditions may not clear up. In such a case, breathing through the mouth is the main choice, and there is no sense in agonizing over it.

Atmosphere

Clearing up every single imaginable interruption, before ruminating, is another fundamental advance. Mood killer, the telephone, eat a little dinner in advance, so you are not only ruminating over being ravenous, and truly set the climate for the reflection session. On the off chance that you practice contemplation after Yoga asana practice, you may have an unfilled stomach, and your session may pursue an inflexible calendar. Never make progress toward flawlessness, since all flawlessness is, at last, a fantasy, yet do what you can to advance a thoughtful climate. Your reflection sessions will improve significantly if you let flawlessness go.

Simple Meditation Techniques and Simple Ways to Practice Meditation

Meditation is the act of utilizing mental meditation and breathing systems to incite smoothness and quietness. Individuals have polished meditation for many years, once in a while as a piece of strict articulation. Be that as it may, reflection isn't restricted to rigorous practice; indeed, a great many people use it just as an approach to adapt to pressure. Figuring out how to ruminate can improve your life and assist you with living every day without limit.

Planning Space for Meditation

It doesn't make a difference where you reflect since you feel loose and quiet. A pleasant spot free of interruptions will enable you to focus. A few people accomplish this by darkening the lights, lighting candles or consuming incense. Others favor a spot where they can feel the glow of the sun. There is no set-in stone spot to reflect, similarly insofar as you're agreeable and ready to center.

Regular individuals reflect in an upright position, sitting with a straight back to encourage profound relaxing. This could mean sitting on the floor or in an agreeable seat. If you intend to sit on the floor, consider getting a yoga tangle for comfort. Oppose the compulsion to rest, particularly in case you're new to contemplation since you'll get drowsy and lazy.

Breathing Techniques for Meditation

Breathing is key to meditation, so it's essential to see how to do it appropriately. To begin with, you ought to sit upstanding with your spine straight. Get settled, close your eyes, and take a full breath until your lungs feel full. You, as a person, need to withhold your very own breath for few seconds at that very point gradually breathe out. Ensure that you inhale through your nose and that you never secure your jaw as you relax.

At the point when you inhale, you should feel your stomach grow forward, and your ribs separate marginally. As you breathe out, attempt and spotlight on the sentiment of air leaving your body. A great many people discover this sensation unwinding, however, be careful with pressure in your shoulder and neck. From the start, it may be difficult to take as such, however with training; it will turn out to be very agreeable.

Quieting your Mind for Meditation

Numerous individuals make some troublesome memories quieting down their psyche from the clamor of the day. Our lives are occupied to the point that the majority of us run throughout the day and break down into bed around evening time. For the day, we consider our work, companions, and family, physical checkups, school, and different commitments we may have. Releasing the entirety of what can be a major challenge.

One strategy you can use to quiet your brain is to just concentrate on the way toward relaxing. This system gives your mind something to focus on, which is more straightforward than attempting to consider nothing by any means. As you inhale, consider the entirety of the sensations you feel. If your mind begins to meander, recognize the idea and refocus on relaxing.

Instructions to Incorporate Meditation into Your Martial Arts Training

Meditation has continuously assumed a significant job in combative techniques preparing. For the individuals who have never attempted to consolidate contemplation into their preparation, consider joining this antiquated system as you learn hand to hand fighting. Numerous experts of various styles propose a particular way contemplate; however, you can utilize any strategy that you are alright with. Meditation, when used during preparation, is a perfect method to help achieve the engaged, quiet mental express that is so critical to acing your battling aptitudes.

CHAPTER 5

A Path Through Meditation

GUIDED MEDITATION SESSIONS

Disclaimer: when listening to meditation recordings, do so in a safe place, preferably where you will not be disturbed for the duration of your recording. Please use your headphones. Never listen to recordings or practice meditation while driving in a car, operating machinery, or doing anything else that requires your attention for safety reasons.

Very Simple and Easy Techniques to Approach Meditation for The First Time with Script

Talking to Oneself

Holding a conversation with you is probably one of the most underrated methods one can use to fall asleep. Most people associate talking to themselves to being given names like 'crazy' or 'geek' but this simple practice can change your sleep patterns for the better.

Insomniacs are good at hurling negative things their own way. Some get to the point of harming themselves because they are so angry with themselves for not being able to sleep. Paradoxically, insomnia tends to feed on the criticism one gives to self. Not everyone gets to the point of inflicting physical harm on himself or herself. Sometimes, the brain fills with negative chatter and questions that only harm sleep progress.

Offer yourself calming words of appreciation and understanding during this time as you talk to yourself. Apply words like "I am sure I can do this" or "It may take some time, but it will work out eventually" or "Everything will be better with persistence." The aim of these positive statements is to reduce any negative feelings and those of anxiety in order to achieve sleep. Negative thoughts will only be a cause for more stress which later builds up to anxiety or even panic attacks.

Mindful Body Scan

This type of meditation is very easy to perform. Conveniently, it can happen as you lie in bed. Rumor has it that it is one of the most popular techniques used by people from the military to achieve sleep.

A body scan involves paying attention to different parts of your body and releasing the tension that has accumulated. A top to bottom approach (or vice versa) usually characterizes it where you can choose to either start from the tip of your head or your feet. The goal is to work your way to the opposite end while releasing tension from each muscle. The duration to do this can vary depending on the severity of the insomnia. Whatever happens, focus on your muscles, and keep releasing the tension.

Use of Mantras

Developing a mantra can act as a good tool to achieve mental clarity while setting your attention on a given phrase. While addressing the issue of mantras, many people form an associative link with yoga and meditation. Actually, they are usable in many more scenarios besides the mentioned ones. The aim of using mantras is to ensure your mind has no room for other thoughts since insomniacs have a tendency of constantly battling fleeting memories.

Even on the occasion that you do not fall asleep, you will be able to notice your mind will be quieter. This means your mind will eventually end up resting in some of its regions giving it a little physical rest. If you are lying comfortably, this will restore your body to some extent.

Although most of the original mantras appeared in Sanskrit, they come in different forms. To keep yourself concentrated, always choose a simple mantra. The following guidelines can help you come up with a good one:

It should be clear with simple wording.

It should be very short to avoid you from thinking about the process.

It should have a calming effect.

It should have an affirmative tone.

When reciting a mantra, your only concern should be saying it internally as you lie down in a comfortable position. Avoid any positions that will lead to twiddling, as this will only reverse your efforts. Try to lie still and breathe deeply as you recite it. Again, if your mind starts racing, refocus your attention back to the mantra.

Visualization

Instead of spending most of your time thinking about your stressful day or your next exam or meeting, try visualization. It can be good practice to help you unwind and fall asleep easily by focusing their attention on calming and soothing images.

Imagine yourself in a place where you experienced a deep sense of calm. Feel free to make your imagination wild. Imagine yourself on your way to that place again and it will be a better experience than you had the previous time. Making your imagination as detailed as possible should be one of your prime goals. What time is it? What kind of clothes are you wearing? What can you see along the way? Keep at it until you sleep.

This method can also be very useful when one decides to use guided meditation. Most scripts require you to imagine a calming scene and if you are good at it, you are halfway there.

Counting Backwards

Counting forward is so easy. You can probably do it while asleep. If counting from 100 seems a bit difficult for you, you can always start from 50 or 70. Make sure you restart when your mind drifts and you lose track. Do not take it too seriously that you beat yourself up when you lose count. This is just a casual exercise. Nobody is watching.

Sleep Hypnosis Script

It is a good idea to familiarize you with sleep hypnosis techniques, considering how important sleep is for our daily functioning. A healthy mind is a wealthy mind. Without a proper good night's sleep, you are bound to run out of energy. Since 50% of the world suffers from insomnia, I would like to share two sleep hypnosis scripts that might come in handy. You can record them in your own voice for personal use when going to sleep.

Script

Lie flat on your back and feel the sensations on your body for a while. Spread your hands and feet comfortably to make sure you are fully relaxed. Now I want you to focus your attention on your breath. I want you to breathe in deeply and fill the bottom of your lungs, causing the lower belly to rise. Hold your breath for a few seconds and slowly release the air while feeling your lower belly drop. Make sure you have emptied every drop of air from your lungs.

Start again by noticing how fresh the air is as you breathe in. Pay attention to filling your lower lungs with air as you feel your stomach rise again. Make sure you have fully filled your lungs with air that you cannot take in more. Pause for a few seconds and let go of the air slowly. Repeat this process seven times. Each time, imagine your body relaxing and letting go of all the tension you have. Let it all fade away as sand washed off by water.

Now, try to feel every bit of your body. Notice any points of tension and just make a note of them. I want you to start relaxing your muscles from the top of your head to your toes.

Tense the crown of your head and release the tension, pushing it to the left side of the head. Tense the left side of your head and release any tension while pushing it to the right side of the head. Do the same for the right side of the head and push the tension to the back of the head. Now, bring your attention to your forehead. Tense your forehead and do away with any tense sensation. If there are still traces of tension, move to the left and right eyebrow. Each time, make sure you tense each part and release the tension, pushing whatever residual tension is left to the next part of the body. Do this twice since is a key area of stress. From your eyebrows, drop down to your nose and tense it making sure to release the tension after a few seconds. Now go to the jaw region and do the same.

Imagine all your tension accumulated in the jaw. Move it down to your neck through your throat. This time too, tense your neck and release the tension twice. When done, you are free to move to your chest region.

From the chest region, repeat the same process, covering each part systematically and not neglecting any region. When you encounter an area with a lot of tension, tense it and release it twice then progress to the other part.

After completing the cycle of the chest and stomach region, transfer your attention to your upper back. Feel any tension present on your left scapula. Your scapula is the bone that is present on the upper back. Tense it and release the tension after a few seconds. Transfer the tension to the right scapula and tense it as well. Release the tension each time making sure to transfer the tension left to the next part of the body. Now continue with the process until you reach your lower back. Make sure to release all the tension or carty the residual to the next part. Now, bring all your tension to the tip of your spine, close to the neck, and imagine it sliding down to join both scapulae and connecting to the shoulders.

Focus on the fingers from the left hand now. Relax and stretch your hand. Tense the muscles in your hand and transfer to your wrist any remaining tension. Add tension then relax, transferring to your forearm the remaining tension. Add tension then relax, and then transfer to your upper arm any remaining tension. Tense, relax, and shift to your shoulder any remaining tension. Repeat the same process for the right hand. When you bring the final tension to your left shoulder, slide both accumulated tensions down to the spine and through the scapulae to the hips.

Tense the hips and relax. Imagine the tension left whirling around in a circle just disbanding itself disappearing. Tense the hips and relax them again. Now, move any tension left in the opposite direction and think of it being washed away by a calming feeling.

Move any residual tension to the thighs. Tense both of them simultaneously and relax. Carry any residual tension to the knees. Tense both of them and relax. Make sure to keep conscious of the moving tension to ensure the previous areas are free of tension. Move down to the shins, tensing them and relaxing them simultaneously after a few seconds. Carry any residual tension to the calves. Tense them and relax them twice. This is a big area of tension. Pay close attention to it as you transfer any residual tension to the ankles. Tense and relax the ankles twice as well. Move to the heels and do the same. Tense and relax them foot by foot. Release all the tension and transfer any left tension to the toes. Imagine all the tension oozing out from the tips of your toes and flowing out of your body. You now feel relaxed and ready to encounter the next journey to sleep.

Now with your completely relaxed body laying still on the bed, feel your body getting lighter and lighter. You can envision yourself floating up and heading for the clouds. You want to go and lay on the cushions of the clouds. Your body, mind, and spirit are calm. You are now in the midst of heavy cushiony clouds. You can feel them comfortably rubbing on your skin as you drift into more cloud comfort. They just keep coming and ones that are more comfortable keep showing up. You can also feel a slight gentle breeze drifting you away. You are relaxed.

MEDITATION FOR BEGINNERS WITH BREATHING EXERCISES SCRIPT

Welcome.

Notice that your eyelids are feeling heavier, they are drooping and closing. Quietness slowly washes over you. It fills your mind and your room. Let it in to soothe you. In the quiet, release all of your stress. Release every worry and give permission to the quietness. Allow yourself, in body and mind, to let go of your anxieties. Allow yourself to be lulled into the calming security of the quiet. You are safe here. Turn your head to one side and feel the muscles in your neck elongate. Return to the center, or a way that feels most natural. Turn your head to the other side and enjoy the stretching of the muscles. Return to the center, or a way that feels most natural. You notice that you are starting to feel more relaxed.

Through your nose, take a deep breath in. Let the breath fill your belly and stretch your abdomen. Hold it in your belly for one, two, three beats and then slowly let it out through your nose. Again, breathe in deeply through your nose filling your belly, and then gently exhale through your nose. Continue to breathe deeply as you slowly shift your focus to the top of your head. From the center of your scalp, a warm sensation unfolds like the petals of a flower in bloom. Slowly, each petal stretches to reveal a bright yellow center. You feel the center of this flower is emanating the warm sensation, a sensation of peace and tranquility. In rivulets, the feeling of calmness trickles down your forehead, over your mouth and chin. It loosens the muscles in your temples and in your jaw, releasing the leftover tension in your face and head from the day. The sensation continues to your neck and shoulders. You feel cleansed by a sense of calm as washes over you. All the tension in your shoulder muscles floats away as the warmth moves forward.

Your arms are now beginning to feel light, too. The warmth travels to your elbows and now your wrists, your hands and now your fingers. Let them feel warm and light, doused in the peace that wishes to engulf you. Let go of the desire to resist the peaceful sensation that washes over you. Embrace serenity with each breath you inhale. Release the control over your body and give into this pleasant, calming sensation.

Breathe in. Now breathe out. Slowly, gently, deeply. Breathe in. Breathe out. That peaceful warmth of relaxation continues to spread. It meanders over each of your ribs, wandering towards your chest. A second flower, bright and red, slowly unfurls to release a second wave of delightful coziness. You feel your chest loosening, opening up to accept positivity. You feel safe, you feel at peace. This sensation roams past your ribcage and into your stomach. This warm feeling calms you, soothes you. As you fill your belly with oxygen, you also fill it with warmth and tranquility and calmness. There is no more room for doubt or worry. You are a being that exists in this world of beauty, not to be bothered by stress. All of your worries begin to fade away into a fine powder or dust that is taken away with the breeze. You let them go, the same way you let go of the muscle tension in your shoulders and your back. You are loosened even more, and you feel light like air.

This feeling moves past your thighs and swims towards the curves of your knees. It continues to travel lower and lower. Notice how your legs are feeling weightless and you are feeling calmer than ever before. There are no worries anymore, only this light and loving warmth. Give yourself over to the sensation that cloaks your body from the toes upwards. Drift into a deeper feeling of serenity and tranquility with every breath that you take.

Continue to breathe deeply as you feel the sensation of quiet warmth glide over your knees and into your calves. The warm sensation fills your ankles and slowly seeps into the soles of your feet and finally descends into the very tips of your toes, warm and cozy beneath your blanket. Gently curl your toes as you feel the warm sensation undulate throughout your body. All the tension in your muscles floats away as the warmth gives way to weightlessness and you feel as though you could float right into the atmosphere.

Realize how freeing it feels to release all your tension. In this very moment nothing else matters. You are free. You are warm. You are weightless. There is nowhere for you to be except here, floating on a cloud of nearing sleep. You have everything you need. You are here, allowing the peaceful sensation to radiate through your body. With each breath you take, you are feeling more and more serene. Breathe into your soul a wealth of peace and harmony. Breathe out, expelling all the leftover negative energy and therefore releasing your control. Realize how good it feels to be so safe and so relaxed.

Your body is light and warm as you listen to my voice. Let me guide you as you drift away. I am now going to count, and you will listen. Let my voice lull you. You are safe and relaxed and warm.

Ten... Your entire body is relaxed. Every muscle has loosened.

Nine... You are surrounded by quietness, stillness, and tranquility.

Eight... You can feel the warmth of those who love you, enveloping your senses.

Seven... You are lulled further into an even deeper state of relaxation.

Six... With each breath, you inhale all of the goodness in the world.

Five... You exhale all of the bad, blowing away all of your stress, your worries, your sorrows, and pain.

Four... You feel your body becoming lighter, weightless, as a feather in a summer breeze.

Three... You feel your mind brimming with warmth and love. The blooming flowers on top of your head and chest reinforce these sensations.

Two... Accept the peace that surrounded you, know it's lovely. Let it send you out into the feeling of relaxation ever deeper.

One... You get as far as you can, higher up into the night sky, with comfort and sleep, rising all the way up.

You are healthy, so relaxed. Let yourself feel comfortable and secure as you float in this place.

You wade across the starlit sky, among celestial bodies of great power and stillness. You are reminded that you are made up of the same matter: power and stillness, undisturbed by anxiety.

You reach your hand into the water and collect a shell. Perhaps it is round and white, or perhaps it is smooth and pink. You swirl it in the small tide pool to wash off the flecks of sand. The granules float back to the bottom and settle in to rejoin their colony. You hold this delicate shell in your palm, gently turning it over to observe it. The shell is light and has been a traveler of the ocean for an endless expanse of time. Your shell has traversed the saltwater waves for millennia and yet found its way to you.

This ancient relic of the sea reminds you of your own existence, delicate yet strong enough to withstand any storm.

Just the sight of this shell washes you in warmth and security. Again, it begins at the top of your head, trickling outwards from the center of your scalp, cascading over your ears and cheeks and down over your shoulders. It pours over your shoulders, down your arms, over your legs and through the tops of your feet. This shell is a comfort to you.

Remember this shell, glimmering in the palm of your hand. Tuck it away in your memory because any time you are feeling even a tiny bit of anxiety or stress that keeps you from sleep, you are going to call upon this shell. When you call on this shell, the stress will vanish into sand, swept away by the ocean. When you call upon this shell, it will invoke this warming peace you feel. It will wash you in relaxation, and lull you into a deep, tranquil sleep.

I am going to count down from five. When I reach one, you are going to completely and intimately embrace the calmness that has engulfed you and surrender to sleep. You will feel yourself drifting into a peaceful and serene rest.

Five... You think of your shell from the tide pool along the shore. Your ancient shell. It melts away every tension left until your body and mind are relaxed. It is beckoning you to sleep.

Four... You feel the warmth of peace move from the top of your head and down your neck. It travels down your shoulders, radiates through your ribcage and stomach, and finally glazes over your legs.

Three... You feel your body becoming heavy and you softly sink in a little deeper to your consciousness. You are protected. You are safe.

Two ... You feel yourself drifting away, like the salt of the sea on the breeze. You float away, quietly into the night.

One ... You are now asleep, resting and at peace.

Breathe in, Breathe out. Breathe in, Breathe out. When you wake, you will be restored and ready to take on the day with newfound energy and confidence. You will be ready to conquer the obstacles of your life now that you have conquered sleep.

USING GUIDED MEDITATION FOR REDUCING ANXIETY AND STRESS

If we really want to quiet our mind and be a more peaceful individual, then it's important that we understand how to relieve that tension within our bodies. This is going to be a body scan meditation that will guide you through how you can best release any tension in your body.

Most body scans will have you start with your head, but we're going to do the opposite. Make sure that you are in a relaxed place with nothing around you. You should be completely at ease with zero distractions. Keep your legs gently stretched out in front of you and your arms placed by your side.

You can have parts of you slightly bent but nothing to where you're going to add extra strain or tension into that part of your body.

Your knees are important and make your legs more usable. You can bend your legs. Without your knees, you wouldn't be able to twist and move your legs so much. These make us flexible.

Move up now to your thighs. These are the big meaty parts of your legs. They will help make sure that you are able to walk around as you wish strongly. You use this part to help kick. It's what you sit on.

It's where you might be able to feel some tension that might travel up to your hips. This kind of stress isn't always noticeable. We don't frequently think about carrying stress and tension within our legs. However, you can still have so much within these body parts and focusing on them makes it easier for you to let go of tension.

Move up now to your stomach. This is where you can also hold a lot of anxiety. We don't realize just how much our stomachs play a role in the feelings that we have, but it really is in charge of a lot. Your stomach is what processes all the nutrients and minerals that you give to it. It helps regulate your hormonal balance which will play directly into the way that you feel emotionally. Let yourself feel some of the tension as it is released through your stomach.

Sometimes we keep our abdomen stiff and filled with anxiety.

It's hard to think about certain things and you might get nervous butterflies which can be felt within your tummy.

Let yourself release the tension in your stomach. This is such an important part of our body that is the home to so many organs. We need to protect it and treat it as such. Let yourself feel tension vanish from your midsection.

On the opposite side is your lower back, this is another place that will hold an incredible amount of tension. Our backs are often mistreated as we are always slouching. What we don't understand is just how much it can be intertwined with our hips and our stomach and the way that we carry anxiety around with us.

Your lower back can be such a sensitive part as well. It holds your spine and so many nerves responsible for transmitting messages throughout your body. This is an important part that we must take care of. Let yourself feel the tension leave your lower back. You can tense for a moment and then simply release as you regulate your breathing. When you tense your back, this helps remind you of just how much tension there might be.

Move up now to your chest. This is the place that holds your heart and your lungs – some of the most important parts of your body.

It's how the blood and the oxygen get regulated throughout the rest of your systems. It's an incredibly important part of your body and the place where we might feel stressed the most beyond just our minds. How often do you feel your heart race as you are nervous about something? Perhaps you experience frequent trouble breathing because you feel so stressed out.

These parts of your body are incredibly important because, without them, nothing else would be able to function.

Consider the way that you might feel stress and anxiety within these parts of your body.

Do you feel sick to your stomach with a rapid heartbeat and quick breathing when you feel something that makes you nervous? Let yourself really feel your breath now. Focus on breathing in through your nose and out through your mouth once again, as we count down from ten.

10... 9... 8... 7... 6... 5... 4... 3... 2... 1

Feel as your heart continues to beat. Notice that it is getting slower and slower the more relaxed you are. Let's start with our hands as well. We can't overlook these important parts of our body. Your hands can hold whatever you want. They can pet your favorite animal, or you could cradle a little baby. Your hands help you write, create, draw, sketch and do anything else that you enjoy doing. You can craft something new, or you can fix a beloved object. You can write a friend a letter, or you can text them something meaningful. Your hands are incredibly powerful. We can't forget the way that we might even feel tension and anxiety within our phalanges.

Let your hands be flat against wherever they are new, whether they're on the bed beside you or you've placed them on top of your stomach.

Just simply stretch your fingers out and feel the tension leaving them. You might not even realize how frequently you hold a fist with your hand. This fist is the ball of anxiety that we have to carry around with us. Keep your hand flat and open and remind yourself that you are peaceful, and you are calm. Nothing and nobody is going to hurt you within this moment. You are perfectly at ease, and you have nothing to worry about. Move upwards to your elbows. Between your hand and your elbow is another important part of your body. This is what supports you when you might be carrying something.

This is the part of our body that we use to wrap around our friends and loved ones as we give them a hug. You can feel the tension within this part of your body.

Put your hand backward now, pointing your fingers towards your arm, and feel the muscle from your wrist to your elbow. So much tension can be held in this but release it and continue to breathe as you allow yourself to become more relaxed, moving upwards to our biceps. All of this is where we are able to support the things that our hands do.

This is where we connect our hands to our mind. That's how we're able to transport messages and find support within these vital parts of our body. Feel the tension be released as you focus on this now. Continue to let the air come in and out of your body. Move up now to your shoulder and your neck. This is probably where you feel an immense amount of tension.

How many times has somebody touched your shoulder only to tell you that you are feeling pretty tense? This is an area that we need to focus on relieving tension from now, let your shoulders become more relaxed. Feel as your chest gets lighter, and you can breathe just a bit easier.

Your neck has so many important muscles, and it protects what your nervous system needs to do and helps connect your brain to the rest of your body.

It's also where the hairs might rise on the back of our neck when you're feeling scared. You might feel fear and tension within your shoulders because you're always prepared. Release this tension now and let yourself really drop your head into the pillow beneath you.

Our heads are so heavy, and we carry so much around with us, but you can feel that tension release and you now move up to your face in this moment. This is where you send so many signals to other people. You're able to smile, cry, grimace, or make other expressions that can sometimes comfort them.

You can show them that you love them and that you are happy whenever you want by using your face. It is where we eat and notice how we breathe. It is how we hear and how we see. Our face and our entire head are so incredibly important, too.

We have to feel the peace travel through this part as we transmit that message to the rest of our body. This is the control center.

This is where we need to ensure that we are releasing tension. Let yourself breathe in and out, in and out. You can do this body scan whenever you feel like you need to create a more peaceful mind. Continue to focus on the way that you might feel certain tension within parts of your body.

Release this tension as you notice it. As we countdown from 20, you will either drift off to sleep or move on to the next meditation.

20…19…18…17…16…15…14…13…12…11…10…9…8…7…6…5…4…3…2…1…

MEDITATION TO OVERCOME PANIC ATTACK

Panic attacks are a severe form of anxiety that makes a victim become so fearful when there is no reason to warrant such behavior. It is characterized by feelings of terror and the victim might think that they are experiencing heart failure or are about to die.

Researchers say that people usually experience a panic attack a couple of times in their lifetime, which is totally normal, considering that each one of us harbors some fears that are known only to us. But then if we develop a tendency of constantly dealing with panic attacks, say on a daily basis, then there's cause for worry.

Symptoms of Panic Attacks:

These are some of the symptoms felt by the victim of a panic attack:

Thunderous Heartbeat

When you have been running for a long distance, you are likely to experience a higher-than-normal heartbeat, and even then, it's quite disturbing. But when it comes to someone who's been seized by a panic attack, they experience a wildly knocking heart that leaves them gasping for air. Their heart knocks so wildly and they feel as though they are about to die. Panic attacks are extremely uncomfortable fear response mechanisms and it's unimaginable what the sufferer goes through on a frequent basis. This wild knocking of their heart interrupts their peace, magnifies their worry and causes their productivity to take a hit.

Feeling of Weakness

Panic attacks are extremely resource intensive. Once a victim has been seized by the wave of a panic attack, they normally go down and lay in a state of weakness, a clear sign of being ovelwhelmed. The wild beating of the heart consumes a lot of energy and makes a person feel as though they are dying. Actually, it takes some amount of time before they fully recover from the attack. It is advisable that the victim gets something nutritious to eat after a panic attack so as to discourage so that they might continue to function in a normal way.

Numbness in The Fingers and Toes

The wave of the panic attack is so dense that it leaves the victim feeling as though their fingers or toes have no blood. The numbness is attributed to a slight glitch in their nerves thanks to the wild knocking of their heart. But of course, they soon regain the full use of both their fingers and toes.

An Impending Sense of Doom

As the victim of the panic attack struggles with the wildly knocking heart, they feel as though something terrible is about to happen. For instance, they might think that they are about to experience a heart attack, or as if they are about to kick the bucket. This is a testament to the intensity of the symptoms of a panic attack.

Sweating

This depends on the physiological makeup of the victim, but it is not uncommon to see beads of perspiration on a victim's face. The very thought they have been close to dying or losing the use of their heart is enough to trigger their sweat. Victims of a panic attack night still sweat at the remembrance of their symptoms.

Chest Pains

Considering the wild beating of their heart during the panic attack, the victim is left nursing massive chest pains as their chest muscles align back together. It takes a while before the chest pain goes away. But the victim is likely to hold their chest all along.

Difficulty in Breathing

When your heart is beating like crazy, and you are feeling as though you are about to die and your chest is engulfed in a blanket of pain, good luck with breathing. The victim usually struggles to get air and it makes the entire scenario even grimmer. Due to their inability to breathe properly, it might bring about a small headache.

No Control

In general terms, this is what victims of panic attacks feel. They cannot seem to understand what's happening. The pain in their chest, the ringing in their ears, and the numbness of their hands, all make them feel as though they have lost control. It's precisely why the victim of a panic attack hardly does anything besides act shocked.

Derealization

Some victims seem to think that whatever they are experiencing is not real. They feel as though they have been put in some other world and this must not be a reality. This goes to show that panic attacks a.re indeed powerful. Such victims are at the highest risk of developing chronic anxiety.

Tips for Dealing with Panic Attacks

Once your body comes down with panic anxiety, you have the heavy task of dealing with the condition the right way.

The response that a victim gives when they face panic attacks is what determines the extent of the injury.

The following tips are designed to help you get through any form of a panic attack.

Knowledge

If you understand what our body is going through, you won't be as freaked as someone who has no idea what's going on. A panic attack is a sign that your body has experienced a threat and it's in survival mode. Most of the time, these "threats" don't warrant the kind of response that the body gives. For instance, if you are a divorcee, and you happen to be strolling down the street on a fine day only to see a man that closely resembles your ex, your mind might overreact to that incident and cause you to experience a panic attack. But if you are aware of what's happening you will be less affected by the incident. Once you realize that you have this condition, it is also important to read up more on it. This will help you understand how panic attacks truly work and how you may minimize the effects and ultimately overcome this condition.

Be Calm

It might seem like an easy thing but when you experience a panic attack you are bound to be anything but calm. The wild knocking of the heart, the ringing sounds inside your head, the impending sense of doom, is enough to reduce you to a nervous wreck. But then panicking about panic attacks can only make the situation worse – not better. You had better realize how to calm your nerves and develop a rigid mindset. It's the only way to emerge unscathed. Considering that the symptoms of a panic attack are quite strong, the victim must be careful to project the right attitude or else it will make it hard for them to overcome this condition.

Know What Triggers Your Panic Attacks

You might not always know what is behind your panic attacks considering that your brain can magnify even the smallest of incidents. But then issues like traumatic thoughts and obsessive thoughts are potential triggers of a panic attack. You must be wary of the various lines of thinking that result in the development of panic attacks. For instance, if you were abused as a child by one of your close relatives, coming across anything that remotely reminds you of that person is enough to send you into a panic attack, but since you know that you might actually report to your brain that it's okay and dissuade yourself from developing a panic attack.

Of course, it's not as easy as it sounds but through practice, one can become perfect at understanding their emotional makeup.

In order to be able to tell what triggers your panic attacks, you must increase your self-awareness. The easiest way of increasing your self-awareness is through paying attention to your internal dialogues. Don't just waltz through incidents but take the time to understand how your mind interprets reality in relation to the emotional scars that you bear.

The worst kind of panic attack is induced by your thoughts, for then you will have a hard time hiding from your thoughts. Ensure that you have a strong sense of self-awareness so that you may be in a position to contain any potential panic attack.

For instance, if you are sitting in your office trying to be productive, and all of a sudden, automatic negative thoughts of relating to your childhood abuse creep up in your mind, instead of just entertaining these thoughts, you might want to walk into another office and share with them what's happening. In that context, your brain is less likely to feel threatened into taking action.

Mindful Breathing

The thing about panic attacks is that they are involuntary. You can only act and hope that your brain won't get to that. However, if your brain decides to activate a panic attack, you are helpless. But then how you behave after experiencing a panic attack is just as important. You don't want to be the type of person that becomes crushed under worry as you remember that you were about to die.

Mindful breathing is one of the ways to calm you down. Mindful breathing is both a therapeutic and relaxation technique. It helps your racing mind to calm down and realize that you are no longer in danger.

Mindful breathing improves the state of your mind and allows you to savor your reality in a more intensive manner.

Conditioning your mind to experience reality as opposed to wandering off to explore your fears and worries is a great way of handling a panic attack. Assuming that you are in an outdoor setting, then thanks to mindful breathing, you are able to savor the beauty of nature, the blueness of the sky, and you appreciate the natural world. This keeps you from entertaining the dangerous thought patterns that trigger panic attacks.

Visualization

Understand that just as your mind can lead you down the dark and horrible path of panic attacks, it can lead you into spears of light and hope.

You just have to know how to rely on your mind in order to achieve the outcome that you want. One of the best ways of relying on your mind to achieve your goal is through visualization.

There are many ultra-successful people that swear by visualization. It helps them put their fears in the backseat and focus on what they want to achieve.

Visualizing is all about calling to mind the exact thing that you want to experience in reality. For instance, if you are a basketball player, one of your important life goals might be getting the ring.

So, when you visualize, you will see yourself staging an exemplary performance and afterward taking the trophy.

Once you have visualized several times of a particular outcome, you will stop falling victim to your fears and you will develop the fortitude to fight for your dreams.

Interestingly, you can use visualization to cure yourself of panic attacks or at least reduce the effects of a panic attack.

Just get into a comfortable position and watch you experiencing various triggers and yet not developing any form of a panic attack.

In order to become really good at nipping in the bud negative incident and thought patterns before they blow into panic attacks, you have to have a great deal of self-awareness.

It is very easy to develop negative habits under the misconception that you are getting away from panic attacks. So, always watch out.

MEDITATION TIPS FOR DAY AND NIGHT

One of the best aspects of meditation is that you can practice whenever works for you. Whether you need a moment during the day or are trying to settle into sleep, there is always time for some meditation.

If you are looking to meditate at night for some deep rest, you are in luck. For most people, they actually struggle to stay awake during their practice because they're so relaxed. That is why I felt it was important to include some tips and tricks to getting back into your day after a good meditation practice. If you are looking to fall asleep, go ahead and try the script below to help settle you in for the night.

The Sleep Countdown

When we focus our minds, it allows us to take thoughts aware that often interfere with falling asleep. Through this meditation, you can learn how to let go of your thoughts instead of dwelling on them. If you are ready to fall asleep for the night, we can begin.

I want you to begin by finding a position you are comfortable sleeping in. If needed, you can always change, but try your best in this moment to not move around too much. Once you are in place, go ahead and take a nice deep breath in. You will want to hold onto this breath for a few moments and gently let it go.

If your body feels tense anywhere, spend a few moments sending your energy to these locations, and focus on relaxing your muscles. Just allow your body to sink into your mattress. Feel how heavy everything is becoming as you get ready to go to bed. Your mind knows it's time to sleep. Your soul knows that it's time to sleep. Allow yourself to relax into this moment.

Now, I would like you to wiggle your toes. Feel how your feet and legs feel and allow them to relax. There is no need to be holding onto tension. You are in a safe zone, and you are looking forward to a long night of deep rest. If you feel like it, try opening and closing your hands. Allow your arms and hands to relax on the mattress. Take a deep breath and relax.

Bring your awareness to your stomach and your chest. Feel how the chest rises and falls with each breath you take. Breathing is becoming slow and natural for you. You may even feel the need to yawn right now. Allow the oxygen to flow in and out of your body with no effort. You can relax. You are nice and calm.

Now, the sleep countdown will begin. With each number you count, allow yourself to relax and drift off toward sleep. I want you to cunt slowly with me and simply count the breaths that you are taking. All I want you to do is focus on the numbers. If any thoughts pop up in the next new moments, allow them to pass without judgment. All that matters is you, your breath, and the numbers. Simply bring your attention back to the numbers, and then we can begin.

We are going to start with the number thirty. As you become mindful of your breath, picture the number thirty in your mind. Breathe in and back out gently. Focus on thirty. Thirty is your only care right now.

Now twenty-nine. Breathe in gently. Twenty-nine. Feel your body sink further into the mattress; everything is calming down around you.

Twenty-eight. You are feeling more and more relaxed. Sleep is waiting to welcome you with warm, open arms.

Twenty-seven.

Twenty-six. Breathe slow. Breathe deep.

Twenty-five. Allow your attention to drift. You are starting to feel sleepy. Twenty-four.

Twenty-three.

Twenty-two.

Focus only on the numbers. Go ahead and count down on your own. Remember to breathe and allow your mind to drift off into sleep. If you lose track of your count, start at thirty again. Count until you drift into sweet sleep and enjoy your rest...

Sleep...

Sleep...

Goodnight.

Tips for Staying Awake During the Day

If you are meditating during the day, the chances are that you will need to stay awake once your practice is complete. Below, you will find some of my favorite tricks to staying awake after you meditate. The more you practice, the easier it will become.

First, it will be vital that you choose a proper meditation location. If you are laying down in bed during meditation, you are just asking to fall asleep during and after your meditation. Instead, you will want to choose a spot on the floor or even a chair to begin your practice in. This will help you refrain from curling up and going right to sleep. As long as you are sitting, you should have a much easier time staying awake.

Another way you can help yourself stay awake during meditation is to repeat words and thoughts to yourself. When you are concentrating, it can help you stay awake. One of the best ways to concentrate is to repeat words to yourself out loud. For example, if you are practicing one of the self-love scripts from before, say your affirmations to yourself. If that doesn't work for you, you can also try counting your breaths out loud.

A third technique I like to use during meditation is to focus on how my body is feeling. In order to stay awake, try to stay aware of how your body is feeling during meditation. You can pay attention to certain aspects such as your body temperature, your thirst level, or your hunger levels. If you meditate on a full stomach, you may be more likely to fall asleep during practice. Instead, try being aware of your body to help keep you awake.

If you are feeling very tired before meditation and you do not want to sleep after, try taking a nap before. If you are feeling that exhausted, perhaps your body is trying to tell you something. You can always try taking a nap and then meditate to bring yourself back into your day; it can be the perfect way to get started again on the right foot.

Finally, I always suggest choosing a time when you are more alert to meditate. A perfect time is in the morning, just after you wake up. Typically, in the morning, we are in routine to get the day started once we wake up. If you have time, take a few moments to meditate. The important factor is choosing a time when you are more alert. Choose a time and learn how to stick with it so you can create a routine.

How to Be Mindful Through the Day

While it may seem like mindfulness during the day is complicated, there are some simple ways for you to carry these lessons into your daily routine. Much like with everything else in our life, it's all about creating a habit.

Below, I will provide you with just some ways you can be mindful throughout the day.

My first tip to you is to practice mindfulness from the moment you wake up to the moment you go to bed. When you wake up and remind yourself to be mindful, it can set the tone for your whole day. If the first thing you do is remind yourself to be mindful, you can increase the likeliness that you will think about it throughout the day. When you are ready to go to bed, remind yourself again to keep the thought in your mind.

Next, you will want to incorporate mindfulness into your daily activities. Too often, we go through our day on autopilot. We get ready for work, get through our workday, come home, and then go to bed. Instead, try to be more mindful of the little moments throughout your day. You can practice as you drive to work or even while you are in the shower. Take a few moments to note how you feel during these seemingly small moments and see how that can change your whole day.

Another way to become more mindful during the day is to allow your mind to wander! Often times, we feel we must be hyper-focused; otherwise, we won't be productive. Honestly, this couldn't be further from the truth. It's healthy to allow your brain to wander every once in a while. If this happens, it's the perfect chance to become mindful as to why it's happening. Perhaps your brain needs a break from thinking for a moment or two. Spend these moments doing a quick body scan and being mindful of relaxing yourself.

One of the best ways to practice mindfulness is to do it while you are waiting for something or someone. In such a busy world, it's easy to become frustrated when we have to actually wait for something whether you are waiting to check out of the store, or you are simply stuck in traffic. While you wait, use this time to practice your mindfulness. You can bring your focus to your breath and begin to calm your mind. Instead of feeling anger in that moment, practice everything you have learned here and allow yourself to relax.

We all know that mindfulness is not a luxury. It's something we all need to work on and practice. As you meditate on a regular basis, becoming mindful will be something that comes much more naturally for you. Remember that you have so much to be grateful for. You have the power over your thoughts; it's up to you to decide how to use your energy. It only takes a few moments to be mindful; you can even give it a try right now!

MEDITATION TO BEOMING TIRED

How Does Your Body Get Tired?

Getting tired after meditation is as a result of the type of meditation you have practiced. You can become drowsy either in the middle of your meditation or at the end of your meditation, which makes you sleep easily. You get tired by overworking yourself, and not sleeping well.

Meditating to Dispel Energy

If you want to be energetic, here is a meditation that can help you. This meditation helps you have great and refreshed energy. This meditation can be done at any time of the day, in the morning, afternoon or night.

Here are a few steps to help you.

- Sit upright, your back must be straight, and your feet should be flat on the ground, your legs can also be cross-legged in a lotus-style pose.
- Bring out your right hand in front of you and hold it out.
- Breathe out through your left nostril, by blocking the right nostril with one of your fingers, repeat the actions with your right nostril, by blocking the left nostril with one of your fingers.
- Focus on breathing out, breathe out, and breathe in back.
- Repeat the breathing process by blocking one of the nostrils with your fingers again.
- Close your eyes, and do not open your eyes until the end of this meditation.
- Feel your body becoming lighter and calmer.
- Imagine that you are listening to the waves of the oceans, or the chirping of the birds in a jungle.
- Say in your mind, "I allow my body and mind to rest as I meditate now."
- Take a deep breath. Breathe in slowly at first, and then gradually increase your breathing.
- Breathe in and out 5 times, allowing your body to feel relaxed and light.
- Ensure that for each breathing process, you hear an audible sound after breathing out.
- Don't force how you feel. Just focus on your body and imagine that you are becoming lighter.
- Feel your skin, legs, and body, having enough oxygen and blood around you.
- Shift your focus to your space and where you are currently.
- Place your attention on the energy you are about to get from nature. Imagine a fresh breeze gently blowing across you, this breeze rolls over you like a ball.
- You feel your head lighter because of the gentle breeze, and then this breeze flows to your arm and then hips and toes.

- You imagine yourself by the riverbank, you can hear the flowing river by your side.
- The river flows and spreads its bank towards you.
- You feel your body come in contact with the river. You feel the tension in your mind released.
- You begin to feel the energy from this space.
- Think of anything that makes you happy or create a new thing that can make you happy.
- Smile when you think of such a thing.
- Take another deep breath, with your eyes still closed.
- Listen to the waves of the river, and gently walk into it.
- Allow your body to enjoy the new environment.
- You can swim if you want, but let your body feel the movement of the flowing river.
- Stay still in the river and keep listening to the waves of the river.
- You can walk out of the river.
- Still in your position, breathe in and out again.
- Stay calm, do not say anything, just listen to the waves of the river and the chirping of the birds.

By the time you are done with this, you are already energized.

Meditation for Tired Hands

- Sit upright and fold your legs into each other, make sure you are in a comfortable position.
- Take a deep breath. Breathe in and out 5 times. Close your eyes.
- Imagine you are standing in front of a wall; place your hands on the wall. Your palm should be on the wall.
- Try twisting your hands around the wall.
- Keep your hands on the wall, you feel tired in your wrist, you feel tightness around your wrist.
- Drop your hands and place them on your lap.
- Breathe slowly, if you feel any pain, note it Be still for 1 minute.
- Take a deep breath.
- Imagine yourself in a stadium, with a ball in your hands. You throw the ball from the center of the field to the goal post.
- You feel your hands-free and released.
- You feel blood flow from your arm down to your elbow, and wrist and fingers.

- You stand and watch how the ball rolls.
- You pick the second ball and throw it with your left hand. You feel your hands released and relaxed.
- You feel the blood flowing through your arms down to your left elbow, wrist, and fingers.
- You feel relaxed and happy; at this point, you can open your eyes.

Meditation for Your Tired Legs

- If you feel tired in your legs after your day, this meditation technique is for you.
- Start by lying down on back, and get settles in.
- Place your two hands on your abdomen and make your shoulder flat.
- Close your eyes now and focus on your body.
- Take a deep breath. Breath in and out two times
- Imagine what happened throughout the day, remember the meeting you had at work, the presentation you did, or interview you had and take another deep breath in and breath out.
- Get your mind settled in, you can talk yourself at this point.
- Take another couple of deep breathing, feel your belly rising and falling.
- Relax your hands, ankles, and toes.
- Take another deep breath and smile widely. Open your eyes now.
- Shift your hands from your abdomen, to place your hands on the floor.
- Patiently place your hands on the floor and make your shoulder relaxed.
- Raise your one leg up towards your chest, and raise the other one after
- Bend both legs through the knee and wrap your hands around your Continue with the deep breathing now, breathe in and out knee.
- Feel your body getting relaxed, your spine, and your waist.
- Tighten your toes and feet and release them after 5 seconds.
- Rock your knee from side to side and draw your feet with your hands closer.
- Massage the toes of your feet and press it gently.

- Take another deep breath and rock your knee side to side. Play with your knee, tap your knee and thigh.
- Take a deep breath in and out.
- Focus on your body and go back to your first position. Lie on your back and return your legs to the floor.
- Breathe in and out, smile at yourself.
- Imagine that you are by a poolside, with your legs and feet inside the pool.
- Rock both legs in the water, playing with it.
- Feel the cool water on your legs and ankles as you play with the water.
- Take a deep breath and enjoy the scent of the freshwater.
- Shift your focus to your body and open your eyes now Massage your ankles, and knees.
- Massage your toes and feel the tightness in your toes reducing.
- Take one more breath in and out.
- Still lying on your back, close your eyes and breathe in and out.
- Return your hands to your abdomen and take another deep breath.
- Place your both hands under your head and gently relax your shoulder.
- Take another deep breath and spread your legs apart from each other.
- End your meditation with a deep breath and sigh heavily after exhalation.

GUIDED MEDITATION FOR SLEEP SCRIPT

As you get ready for bed, it is vital that you quiet your mind and quiet your body. While it can be easy to lay down and replay your whole day or worry about what the next day holds, this is where mindfulness comes into play. Remember that you are in control of your thoughts and your actions. Sleep time is for resting your mind and relaxing your body. You can set yourself up for success through breathing and meditation. If you are ready to go to bed, work through the following scripts, and enjoy a deep and restful night of sleep.

Relaxing into Sleep Meditation

For these next few moments, I want you to settle yourself into bed. Now that it is time to sleep, I invite you to say goodnight to your loved ones, shut down the laptop, turn off the phone, and set yourself up for success. From this moment on, there is no need to worry about anything that happened today or will happen tomorrow. It is time to be present in this moment and allow yourself the time to settle into a full, restful night of sleep. You deserve this. Go ahead and get comfortable in bed.

Now that you are ready for bed, I want you to yawn. As you yawn, take a nice deep breath in and become mindful of slowing down your breathing. As you exhale, feel as if your body begins to relax into your bed. It may feel silly at first, but yawning allows oxygen to enter your system and lengthen the muscles in your jaw all at the same time.

~~

Go ahead and try to yawn again. Allow for your mouth to open wide and let that yawn out with a long sigh. If you want, you can gently stretch your arms above your head and yawn again. Stretch your arms gently and feel the relaxing pull along your shoulder and back muscles. You may notice that there is tension here, and that is perfectly okay. Allow any judgmental thoughts to pass through your mind and spend some time releasing the tension from these areas with each breath you take.

~~

As your body begins to relax under your blankets, continue to focus on your breathing. In the next few moments, I would like to work on quieting your mind. When it comes to falling asleep, it can be hard for some of us to stop our thoughts. Our minds are going every single minute of the day, getting tasks done, staying organized, and keeping you on track. While this is very helpful throughout the day, it is now time to quiet your mind and focus on getting to sleep. If you feel comfortable with it, I would like to work through some guided imagery to help your mind relax. Remember that at this moment, there is nothing to worry about. All I want you to do is focus on slowing your breathing, allow your body to relax, and softly listen to these words.

~~

If you would like, I now invite you to close your eyes gently. As you begin to find your peace, begin to form an image in your head. I want you to begin to picture a comfortable room that is dark. This is a comfortable darkness where you feel safe and warm. As you settle in here, begin to picture a candle sitting in front of you. The candle is glowing warm and flickering gently around you. Go ahead and breathe as you watch the light from the candle dancing across the wall and the floor around you.

~~

As you look at this candle, feel yourself relaxing into the patterns of the light. The soft light relaxes your mind and relaxes your body. Imagine now that your tension and stress are melting away like the wax on the candle. As it burns, feel as the relaxation washes over the crown of your head to the tips of your toes. Allow yourself to gently ease into a deep rest as you watch the candle. Feel yourself melting away, completely relaxing in your bed, your thoughts slowing, and your eyes becoming heavier with sleep. Take a few deep breaths in your own time and allow the sleepiness to take over your mind. When you are ready to fall asleep, blow out the mental candle, and simmer in the new sensation of relaxation.

Meditation Time: **10 Minutes**

Sleep Body Scan Meditation

Now that your mind is rested, it is time to take a few moments to relax your muscles. By getting rid of some of that final tension, you will wake up tomorrow morning feeling well-rested and energetic. In the next few moments, we will work together to release the tension that typically builds in a few focused areas. As you hit the reset button, your body will be able to rest fully and be ready for tomorrow with full strength.

~~

In the following meditation, I am going to invite you to tense and relax each muscle. When you tense the area mentioned, it is vital that you never feel pain as you complete each task. If you feel any discomfort, discontinue this meditation and continue on to the final meditation for the night. This is meant to benefit you, not harm you. When you are ready to begin, take a deep breath, and we can get started.

~~

Now that you are settled in bed take a few moments now to take note of how you feel. There is no need to change anything right now. All I want is for you to be aware of your own body and where you hold onto your tension. There is no right or wrong when it comes to this task, just be mindful.

~~

To begin this exercise, we are going to start with your shoulders and your neck. These two areas are pretty common to hold your stress. When you think about it, many of us work desk jobs and spend the whole day typing. It is all too easy to hold our shoulders up close to our ears and build up the tension. Right now, I invite you to create this movement on purpose. Go ahead and gently raise your shoulders up to your ears and tighten your muscles. As you hold this position, feel how the tension builds up. After a few beats, release and allow for your shoulders to drop back into a comfortable position. Do you feel how much better this sensation is? Now that you are aware, you can practice throughout the day. Go ahead and do this again. Take a few deep breaths and let all of the tension here go for the night. Feel how wonderful it is to relax your neck and settle into the comfort of your pillow.

~~

With your neck and shoulders relaxed, I would now like to bring your focus up to your head. Let's go ahead and start out with your forehead. First, gently raise your eyebrows. As you do this, become mindful how the tension that is created in your forehead. Now, scrunch your eyes closed and furrow your eyebrows. When we are frustrated or stressed, you do this without even thinking about it. As you move through raising and furrowing your eyebrows, take note of how this tension feels. When you are ready, allow your eyebrows to return to a neutral position and allow for your forehead to relax completely. Breathe and relax. You are doing a wonderful job.

~~

When you are ready, slowly bring your focus down to your jaw. Before we do anything, what position is your jaw in right now? Is there tension here? Are your teeth clamped together? If they are, this is okay. The point is being aware. If you are tense here, it is time to relax and let that tension go.

~~

To start off, clamp your jaw shut even tighter. Your lips should feel tight and tense across your teeth as you complete this action. Hold... and then relax. Allow all of the tension to leave your mouth and let your jaw fall loose. Breathe deep and enjoy the comfort of letting this tension go. Throughout the day, many of us clamp our jaws without even realizing it. As you lay here in bed, gently wiggle your jaw back and forth and let go of any lingering tension. Take a deep breath and allow yourself to settle into bed even further. As you relax, your eyes will probably begin to feel heavier. This is your body accepting the relaxation. You deserve a full night of sleep. Allow for this to happen naturally. Take a deep breath and let it all go.

~~

For these next few moments, I just want you to focus on your breathing. As you become mindful of your breath, gently slow it down. Breathe deep through your mouth and hold the air in your lungs for a few beats. Do this again in your own time, and just concentrate on how this breathing makes you feel.

~~

Now that your mind and your body are relaxed, it is time to move onto our final meditation for the night. Your body should be loose, and your mind should be at peace. If not, take a few more moments to settle into your practice and just breathe until you feel okay. When you are ready, we will move onto the sleep count down so you can settle into a nice, deep sleep for the night.

Meditation Time: **15 Minutes**

GUIDED MEDITATION FOR INDUCING SLEEP

Put yourself in a physical position where you can easily fall asleep.

There is a strong possibility that you are already feeling the urge to sleep.

If you are there right now, give yourself permission to do so.

If you are not feeling sleepy, go ahead and close your eyes anyway.

This is the first step to entering into the place of rest.

Keep your focus on the sound of my voice.

This is a good time to remind yourself that even as you enter into this hypnotic trance that leads you to sleep, if there is anything that requires your immediate attention in the world outside your bed, you will immediately snap out of your sleep trance and become alert to your environment.

No matter how deeply you fall asleep, you can still revert to your alert state if the need calls for it.

Keep your breathing slow and regular.

In your thoughts repeat this mantra "I am there already to embrace sleep".

If a thought keeps persisting even after all the exercises you have done, do not give it to him. Simply remind yourself that you will attend to the thought when you wake up.

No matter how pressing a thought maybe, priority at this moment is your sleep.

Now take a deep breath and count back from 20.

When you get to one, shift your focus to your body.

Picture yourself as you lie down where you are.

Do not open your eyes. Rather, see yourself with your inner eye.

Experience your body from the inside.

Now take a slow, deep and cleansing breath. Inhale deeply and exhale slowly

Feel your body rise and fall in rhythm with these breaths that you take.

On each exhale feel the muscles of your body relaxing.

Take another deep and cleansing breath.

Then picture your body drifting away slowly.

There is no sense of direction. No sense of time.

You are just floating away into your subconscious.

Your body is as light as a feather, both physically and mentally. There is nothing holding you back. You are free.

Tune out any other sounds that threaten to invade this subconscious meditation.

Use my voice as an anchor.

You are at peace with yourself and with the universe.

Your mind is clear as the sky on a sunny day.

Your body is continuously drifting and as this happens, feel your breathing slow down even further.

Your eyelids are becoming heavier.

You are not struggling with this feeling.

Just as you drift into this delightsome abyss without resistance, you are also embracing these signs of sleep without fighting them.

There is no need to fight off sleep.

You will wake up in a few hours feeling refreshed and revived.

Your life is colorful and even though there are pressing things that may threaten to take your attention, remind yourself that this moment right here is a priority.

Remind yourself that your body is responding to its biological need.

In the subsequent meditations that you will carry out after this one, when you get to this part, keep your focus on my voice alone.

Do the best you can to ignore everything that 1s happening m your environment.

If this is your first attempt at meditation, try not to worry about the fact that you can still hear those sounds or that those sounds are still able to distract you.

This is a process that will be mastered over time.

But until then focus on the sound of my voice and the rhythm of your breathing.

You are a glorious creature; fearfully and wonderfully made.

Your mind is one of the most intricate aspects of your being.

There is nothing to worry about in terms of how you feel right now.

You are on a journey to self-discovery and while the process may not play out the way you want it, the result remains the same.

You are entering into a place of rest. Your body and mind are in harmony.

There are no distractions to keep you from experiencing healing sleep.

In the next few minutes, you will not just fall asleep, you will fall into a deep and restorative sleep.

So that by the time you get up, whether it is in the morning or in the hours leading up to your shift, you are ready to take on the day.

Sleep will restore you from the crown of your head to the sole of your feet.

In this sleep, you will be able to reconcile the emotions and feelings that have troubled you over time and kept you from sleeping.

Instead of becoming controlled by them, you will learn how to control them.

The truth is that your emotions are there to alert you to the events unfolding in your environment.

They are not meant to dictate your actions.

They do not necessarily mean that you have to act on them.

They are simply there to connect you to the true intent of your heart.

As you successfully induce yourself into a sleep trance, your mind and body ties are temporarily separated.

You do not respond physically to the contents of your mind unless it has to do with sleep.

In the same way, your mind does not hold your body back. Not unless it is protecting you from anything that will prevent you from sleeping.

In this moment, all that matters is the experience of sleep. You are now ready to fall asleep.

Keep breathing slowly and deliberately Keep drifting away mentally.

You are one step closer to your sleep goals.

DEEP SLEEP MEDITATION

Good evening and welcome to this guided deep sleep meditation. In this meditation, you will take some time to go a journey on a path to a deep state of relaxation. You will experience a wonderful calmness and meditative state of mind.

This time is for you, and you are alone. You do not need to do anything. You are completely in control of this meditation session, so you can return to your awakened state whenever you wish. You can do so by just opening your eyes once more.

Simply allow yourself to relax and choose to give yourself this time to unwind and sink deeper into the state of relaxation. Let us start with a simple breathing exercise to help relax the body and mind. No need to close your eyes yet. You want to create a natural breathing rhythm first before you start to really get into meditation.

So, take 3 deep breaths from the diaphragm now.

In...

And out...

In... And out...

In... And out...

Excellent. Now, allow your eyes to close comfortably. Relax your body and let your body be supported by whatever is underneath you. Lean back into this support. Right now, there is nothing you need to do other than focus on your breathing.

Take it nice and easy and let your body loosen up. Continue to breathe as you were and let your body sink deeper into this state of relaxation.

~~

You are grounded in the present moment. It accepts you exactly as you are right now. Feel the surface beneath your body. Surrender any holdings to it. Exhale, and let any tension flow out of you, out of your mind, out of your body and allow a space to open up around you that's just for you.

Continue to breathe deeply from the diaphragm for another while to let your body loosen up and sink deeper into relaxation.

Now, breathe in deeply and exhale fully.

Breathe in deeply...

And exhale fully...

Allow the sound of your breathing to soothe and calm your mind and soul.

Breathe in deeply...

And exhale fully...

Let us proceed with a body scan exercise. To have a restful sleep, one needs to have a relaxed body and mind. You can do both with deep breathing. Start breathing deep and slowly intentionally to take in the air and all its healing energy. Choose to let your body harness this energy to heal, to rejuvenate, after a long day of work.

Scan your body for any areas of discomfort. As you notice any discomfort, begin to give that sense of discomfort a color, a shape, or a texture. Use the power of your imagination to visualize and materialize this discomfort.

Try not to hold any parts of your body in any position... Relax and let them fall into their natural resting position... Maintain your deep and slow breathing... Let your breath soften up your tense muscles as you breathe slowly and deeply...

Continue these deep breaths, making sure to fill your lungs and breathe deep into your belly.

As you breathe in, feel the positive energy flowing into your body. As you breathe out, visualize the negative energy, stress, and worries flowing out of you.

Now, bring your attention to your toes. Wiggle your toes and feel where they are tense or sore. If you notice any tension in your toes let it melt away.

Now bring your attention to your feet. Wiggle your feet a little bit. Tense and flex the muscles in your feet as tightly as you can and then let it go. Feel the tension in your feet melt away and allow them to relax.

Next, let's bring our attention to your ankles. Move your feet around a little to engage your ankles. Then allow them to relax as much as possible. Scan your ankles for any points of tension and just let it all melt away.

Now focus on your calf muscles on the bottom half of your legs. Squeeze your calf muscles tightly and then let go. Relax completely and let all the tension in your legs melt away.

Next focus on your knees. Is there any soreness or tension in your knees? Where are they sore? Now, tense your body as tightly as you possibly can and hold, before completely releasing and relaxing your whole body.

Clenched every muscle tightly...

And relax, letting go...

And again, tense your body as tightly as you can.

Tighten your body as if you are squeezing out all the tension from your body...

And relax, letting go now of all the tension and completely relaxing your body...

For the final time, tense your body as tightly as you can...

Squeeze every muscle as hard as you can...

And relax... letting go now of all the tension and completely relaxing your body.

Where are they tense? Visualize yourself sending yourself healing white energy to your knees. Your body is designed to heal itself. Let your knees completely relax.

Now focus on the upper half of your legs. Without moving your legs too much, tense up your upper leg muscles and then relax them and let go. Feel the tension you keep in your legs melt away and become fully relaxed.

Now bring your attention to your pelvic area. Feel where your body is sitting or lying. Feel where your pelvis touches the seat or where it touches where you are lying. Scan for areas of tension or discomfort.

Visualize your body sending healing white light to any areas that are holding tension and stress.

Feel your muscles relax and your tension starts to drift away.

Now bring your attention to your lower back. Many of us carry around tension in our lower backs. Where do you feel pain? Visualize yourself sending healing energy to these areas and feel the tension melting away.

Next move your attention to the front of your body, your stomach. Feel your stomach rise and fall as you breathe in and out. Our stomachs are often where we feel things first, this is why we say things like "I have a gut feeling this is a good or bad idea.

It's also why we often get indigestion or nausea when we are dealing with highly stressful events. Allow your stomach to relax. Feel all of the tension you hold in this area drifting away.

Now move your attention up to your chest, your heart. Feel your chest rise and fall as you breathe in and out.

Maybe you can feel or hear your heart beating. Allow yourself to experience this fully. As you breathe out release all tension and stress.

Next, pay attention to your upper back behind your chest. Whether you're sitting or lying down feel the area where your upper back makes contact with the surface behind you.

Our upper back suffers a lot from both the stress we carry and our long hours sitting at work, often typing on computers. Feel your breath enter your body and your ribs expand.

Breathe out all of the tension and stress in your back and completely relax.

Now move your attention to your shoulders, another great area for storing stress. This is why we say we feel like we are carrying the weight of the world on our shoulders.

Do you do this too? Are your shoulders flexed to bring them towards your ears? Release this and let them move away from your ears.

Feel all the stress and tension released, as it slowly drifts away. Now bring your attention to your neck. Where does your neck feel sore or tense? Where are you holding onto tension?

As you breathe out, allow all of the tension and stress in your neck to be released. Now move your attention to your face. Let your mouth and cheeks relax.

Squint up your face as hard as you can and then let it all go. Relax your face muscles and let the tension melt away. Move your attention now to your eyes and forehead, where are you holding tension here?

Feel this tension melt away as you begin to relax fully. Lastly, bring your attention to the top and back of your head. Is there any tension here? As you breathe out, breathe out all of the tension. By now you should be fully relaxed. Take a moment to enjoy this pleasant sensation.

As you take a gentle inhale and exhale you realize that the boat has started to move again slowly across the gentle ocean to take you back right where we started the boat has bumped up against the pier you feel completely relaxed.

Any tension in pain you had noticed before is gone. You were quite excited and happy that your shoulders are relaxed that your back feels loose straight and strong.

You notice that your hips feel open and supported, and all tension in your legs and feet have been released. With a joyous inhale, you stand up and carefully walk to the edge of the pier and with complete intention and completion, having received everything that you needed in the amounts that you needed it.

Now, as you find yourself feeling more and more relaxed, start counting down from 5 to 1. As you count each number, you will feel more and more relaxed until you reach a sense of complete and wonderful relaxation.

5... Feeling more relaxed...

4... Allowing the sound of your breathing to calm your mind...

3... Comfortably relaxed,

2... So deeply relaxed ...

1... Your mind is now calm.

Allow the sound of your breathing to continue relaxing your whole body and take your time to enjoy this wonderful experience. You can remain in this deeply relaxed state for a while and smile as you now have completed this meditation session. You can now have a restful sleep.

GUIDED MEDITATION THAT PREVENTS YOU FROM FEELING DRAINED AND TIRED IN THE MORNING

Whether you are feeling overwhelmed with the stress of day-to-day life or suffer from insomnia, falling asleep may not be as simple as lying down and closing your eyes. Too many stressful thoughts and distractions can interfere with your ability to give your body the rest it needs. Self-hypnosis is an effective aid for getting to sleep sooner and staying asleep all night. Try these simple breathing techniques and sleep hypnosis to maintain your calmness throughout your sleep and your life.

Pick a tranquil moment

Locate an agreeable, calm spot to sit or rest

Turn off telephones and request that the family and friends to not to disturb you

Take your place

You can do this practice sitting or lying down

Stay in completely relaxed manner

Don't do anything immediately Ground yourself first

Just sit or lie down completely relaxed for a few minutes

Get into a comfortable position

Keep your back straight

Ensure that your shoulders are also straight

Your back and neck should be in a straight line

Now, gently close your eyes

Notice if there is tension anywhere in your body

If you feel any part tense, release the tension

Adjust your body to release the pressure

Start by breathing normally

Inhale

Exhale

Don't try to increase or decrease the rate of your breathing

Just focus on your breathing

Inhale

Exhale

Inhale

Exhale

Now take a moderate, full breath Inhale gradually through your nose

1... 2... 3... 4...

Hold your breath for a second or two

Gradually exhale through your mouth

4... 3... 2... 1...

Take a deep breath through your nose

1... 2... 3... 4...

Hold it

Breathe out through your mouth

4... 3... 2... 1...

Again, inhale gradually through your nose

1... 2... 3... 4...

Hold your breath

Gradually exhale through your mouth

4... 3... 2... 1...

Now while you are breathing deeply

Say to yourself these simple hypnoses:

From now on, each night

Night after night

As I prepare to go to bed

I will have a feeling of calmness and preparedness for sleep

And I will be able to feel completely relaxed

And at ease

Feeling calmly relaxed

Knowing that every day is another day complete

And knowing tomorrow I will experience new challenges

From now on

As I prepare to go to sleep every night, I will be calm

More and more calm

Every night, and at ease

More and more at ease

My mind and my body will be released

Relaxed

Rested

I will be able to sleep with tranquility, confidence, deeply, securely

Free, and at peace

Sleep the best I have ever had

Sleep as I did as a small child, as a baby, undisturbed, settled deep

Totally fallen into a deep sleep, calmly deeply relaxed

Able to use all the usual noises of the world to soothe my sleep deeply

Totally at peace

I will allow my imagination and creativity to offer a deep and undisturbed calmness

A restful calmness

A deep and restful calmness

Completely rested

From now on I will sleep soundly

So soundly

Knowing in the back of my mind, that day by day

I am beginning to sleep more fully, more deeply

I will sleep wonderfully easily

Restfully

Very easily

Very restfully with a depth and calmness just right for you

Waking at the right time to start your day

As I wake in the morning

I will wake from a deep, restful, relaxing, calm, sleep

Feel fully satisfied from my deep restorative sleep

Feel refreshed, very well, and very calm

And when I wake up in the morning

I will be completely refreshed and totally energized

This will happen just as I say it will happen

When I prepare for sleep, I will feel ready to sleep

I will go to bed with a feeling of calmness and preparedness for sleep

And I will be able to feel completely relaxed and at ease, feeling calmly relaxed

So, starting now, I will go to bed, ready to have deep sleep

And I will enjoy that deep sleep, knowing I will sleep like a baby

Every night, I will be calm

At ease, my mind and my body will be calm, tranquil and relaxed

I will be able to sleep calmly, soundly, securely, at peace

Able to sleep the way I did when I was a baby

So relaxed, so untroubled, so calm, so completely at peace.

NAPPING MEDITATION

Sometimes, you don't always want to fall into a deep sleep, but you still wish to nap in order to get some extra rest. You need to focus on counting to make it happen. Nonetheless, even if you don't drift off in the process, that is fine. All that matters is that you are relaxing.

Aside from visualizing each number as you do a mental countdown, you will also want to picture yourself in extremely relaxing settings. You can be on a vacation, for instance. You can envision yourself on a beach, right by the ocean. Likewise, you may see yourself in a room that you really love. It does not matter if it is a place that you have actually been to or not. It does not have to exist either physically.

Another image that you can hold on to is of you taking a stroll in the mountains. You can also envision yourself in a fancy Italian restaurant or a pink or blue party room with confetti, balloons, lots of joy, and children laughing or any place that makes you feel peaceful. That is the thing - you want to be in a setting that exudes tranquility.

In this process, you may find yourself remembering the details of your day, even the unpleasant parts. Do not fight those images that may come to you, no matter how unsettling they may be. Allow each one of them to pass. Fighting such ideas will only bring on stress, which will defeat the purpose of relaxation. That is not what you want to happen. Let all the good and bad images come and go, and you will see that everything will eventually pass. That is a promise. Once that takes place, then you can be on your way to relaxation again.

And when you are back to this resting mode, you can envision anything that brings you peace. Yes, you can envision animals or going on an African safari as well if the thought makes you feel serene. You can even think of going on the tour physically. You are in the back of the moving safari truck, looking at the pride of lions while the lionesses are caressing their young. You can see the buffalo grazing in an area, as well as a group of zebras running in the distance. Any peaceful image is acceptable.

Meditation for Napping

This meditation is considered as one of the shortest practices because it should be used only when you are trying to nap. If you are not aware of it yet, there is a difference between sleeping and napping. Both have their respective benefits, but this technique is most helpful when you want to doze off quickly and get the burst of energy that will allow you to carry out other tasks during the day.

Before you start, ensure that you are in a safe place to nap. Set your alarm clock properly as well because it is possible for you to fall into a deeper sleep while napping. Try this meditation for the first time when you have time to rest longer to figure out how well you react to the practice. Make sure that you are comfortable and ready to get anywhere from 20 minutes to an hour and a half of sleep. Otherwise, you may not get the desired effects from this napping meditation. Moreover, we are going to use the visualization method for this process. If you do not fall asleep all the way, that is fine. What is most important is that you are allowing your body to rest until you feel rejuvenated.

Assuming that you are already laying on a comfortable mattress or bed, place both of your hands on your stomach. Let your palms touch your abdomen so that you can feel the air as it comes in and out of your body. The air is not exactly in your stomach, but your diaphragm will expand as your lungs get filled with it.

Begin by breathing in slowly through your nose. Allow yourself to draw as much air as possible before letting it out as slowly as you can through the mouth. Doing this too fast can make your heartbeat speed up and keep you awake.

I am going to count down from 20. Each thought you have that does not help you to take a nap, you should push it out of your brain. Concentrate on making sure that you are centered in the present. When I reach one, you are going to think of nothing else other than your slumber. Continue to breathe in as deep as physically possible and release the air as much as you can.

As you feel your eyes grow tired, and your lids start to shield them, think of the darkness. By doing so, you can feel your breathing. You hear nothing but the white noise that surrounds you. While relaxing, you also start to see a tiny white light ahead of you. You walk towards this white light, realizing that it is a door to the outside world.

You step through that door and see that there is only a hot tub in front of you. As you look forward, there is a great view of the blue sky and a beach with white sand waiting for you. The hot tub sits alone on a crisp wooden deck, and nothing else surrounds it. You look down at yourself and notice that you are already wearing your bathing suit, ready to walk into the water.

You slowly start to move towards the tub. It is completely clean and looks as though it has been prepared just for you. There is not another soul around you, and you have the luxury to relax in this warm pool completely.

You take one step in, feeling the warmth of the water engulf your leg. You dip the other leg as well, letting your body acclimate to the new temperature. The water begins to creep up around you, too, making the rest of your system feel as warm as your toes are now.

The level of water comes up over your waist, reaching your arms and shoulders like a soothing blanket. You sit back in the tub and let the jets hit your body. They are pushing all of the tension out of you and releasing them into the water.

You feel yourself drifting off in that cozy tub, but you are still slightly aware of your surroundings. You have no intention of falling asleep completely because you do not want to spend too much time in the water. This simple dip is enough to relax you.

Your eyes close, and you can feel your body loosen up. The sound of the jets soothes you, and your face gets filled with color, it isn't cold or hot outside, but in this tub, you are completely warm.

You feel light as you float there in the water. You aren't moving and can stay grounded in a seat, but you have the ability to feel the weight of your body drift to the top. This makes you feel free and totally at ease.

You think of the times when you were a child, and bath time used to be an entertaining event. The warm water would sometimes scare you, but now you embrace it. Even when the water is a little too hot, it still invigorates your tired body.

Getting out of the tub can be a little challenging at this point, but that's alright. Your face is starting to get hot anyway. If you stay for too long, your skin will be prune-like, and then you may become too used to the temperature.

You are not focused on what is about to happen. The only thing that matters is that you are relaxing in this instant. Your eyelids close again, even though you know that it is almost time to get out of the hot tub. That, too, does not matter at the moment. You merely concentrate on the peacefulness of your surroundings.

The longer you stay in the tub, the more tired you grow. It is time to get out soon, but that is still up to you to decide.

Now, we are going to end the meditation. You can either fall asleep or allow this to be your resting period before waking up and carrying on with the day. When I count to ten, you are going to be completely rested. Continue to feel your breathing with your hands on your stomach and try to keep every part of your body in a relaxed state.

Meditation for A Quick Burst of Energy

Once you have finished napping, you know that you have to wake up so that you can head back to work, school or any activity that has made you tired in the first place. So, it will be beneficial to do this quick meditation that will help you to snap back into reality after a power nap.

Start by closing your eyes as hard as you can in order to feel the muscles in that area tense up. Hold them like that as you breathe in for the first five counts, and then out for the last five.

Relax your eyes now but ensure that your eyelids are still closed.

Now, it is time for you to open your eyes. Pick one thing in the room where you are and stare straight ahead at it. Make sure that the object is directly in your line of vision. Once again, we are going to breathe in 10 times.

Close your eyes and breathe normally for just a moment. When I count to three, snap your eyes open. This time, however, do not look straight ahead. Instead, gaze into your eyelids as high as possible so that you don't see much other than black. Never strain your eyes to the point that it hurts, though. Hold this stare for three counts, and on the third, snap your fingers together and look straight ahead. You will then be alert.

On the count of three, look up. One, two, three. Now, hold this for one, two, three.

Snap and look ahead. You should now feel refreshed. Repeat the steps as needed to be able to wake up completely after a nap or even a night of deep sleep.

MEDITATION FOR SPIRITUAL CLEANING

This final meditation is one that is going to teach you how you can go through spiritual cleansing. This is going to be a method that will help cleanse you and your thoughts. We have provided you with the right mindset tools needed for you to heal from anything that might have happened while preparing for greater challenges as well.

Spiritual Cleansing Meditation

We often pay attention to how we can heal our minds or our bodies, but we need to remember to heal our spirit as well. Spiritual cleansing doesn't have to be about some mystical voodoo magic that is unexplained. Your spirit is a part of you; it is who you are. It is the character that you have built. It is what you believe, it is your virtue. It is your dedication and passion.

Your spirit is a part of who you are, and we need to figure out how to heal it. We are going to take you through the steps of spiritual cleansing. This is something you can do daily, weekly, or monthly. As long as you are dedicating time to cleansing your spirit, you will notice the many benefits of this meditation practice.

Start first by going to a place where you can completely shut out and relax. Free yourself of all distractions.

Begin by breathing in, for five, four, three, two, one, and out for one, two, three, four, and five. Again, breathe in for five, four, three, two, one, and out for one, two, three, four, five.

Continue this as we take you through the journey of spiritual healing. First, we need to learn how to appreciate our bodies.

Our bodies are the spiritual vessels that we interact with throughout the world. Your body helps carry you throughout your day-to-day life. Your body is like a tool that our spirit needs in order to thrive and survive.

Begin to appreciate your body.

Start from the very top of your head and work your way all the way down to the tips of your toes. Breathe in for five, four, three, two, one and out for one, two, three, four, five. Notice now how connected you feel to your body as you start to breathe.

You can feel the air as it fills every last part of your body. The place that needs the air the most is your brain. This is at the very top of your head. Your brain holds together your spirit and your mind.

Your spirit is who you are. It is how you think that makes you a unique individual person. It is the way that you are able to love and understand others, which creates a unique character within yourself. Your spirit is somebody strong and passionate. Your spirit helps you find your motivation and your dedication.

Thank yourself. Give gratitude to this incredible brain that we have. Even when it might not think something that we want or might cause us to say something that we don't even mean, we still have to appreciate all the good that our brain can do for us. Begin to work your way down now to your face. This is how you tell others what your spirit is feeling. You can smile. You can cry. You can laugh. You can show anger, interest, intrigue, or curiosity.

Your face is an incredible tool that your spirit uses to share a message. We can use our mouth to talk, our mouth to eat, and our mouth to breathe. This is so powerful, all in one tiny spot on your entire body. Feel this part of you now as you relax further and further. Feel how the air coming into your body fills you with everything needed to feel better. Allow this meditation to be one where you are saying thanks to your body. Appreciate each little vessel that we discuss.

Your eyes are able to see so much. You can pick up on things around you that others might not even see. You're able to use your eyes to discover the things that you love. Your eyes help you see the people that you care about most. They make you a strong person who's able to complete tasks efficiently.

Move down now to your ears. Your ears can help you hear and understand everything that's around you. You have no problem hearing all that's important. Your ears allow you to hear fun and exciting news. You can hear music and movies that you enjoy and love watching. Your ears are incredibly powerful.

Move down to your shoulders. Your shoulders are what can connect your arms to the rest of your body. These arms are so powerful. They can carry and hold loved ones. They can help you lift things up when needed. You can create with these arms and these hands. Your fingers can touch, and they give you greater insight into what things you enjoy. You can make food and other people happy all by using your hands. You can touch somebody's face and let them know that you're close to them. You can rub their back and make them feel better. You can hold and embrace them so that they don't feel scared or alone.

Breathe in and feel the air travel through these parts of your body. Allow yourself to find a deeper connection to your arms and your hands. Allow yourself to relax these parts of your body.

Move to your chest. Your chest is where your heart beats. The beating of your heart can tell you how you feel. When it's rapid and quick, it tells you that you're scared or worried. When it's slow and heavy, it's nice and relaxing. Close to your heart are your lungs. Breathe in again now and feel as if your body fills with air.

Breathe in for one, two, three, four, and five, and out for five, four, three, two, and one. Feel this incredible strength as it travels in and out. You are capable of everything, because of your heart, your lungs, and your brain. You can accomplish anything that you need to feel better in this life. Move down now to your stomach. Your stomach can tell you so much. It gives you an intuition. You have a gut feeling that can make it easier for you to decide what might be good for you and what might not be in any given situation. This is your power. It's what makes you capable of anything in this world. You are incredibly strong. You have all it takes to heal your spirit.

Now let's remind ourselves of how this body can connect us to the earth. The earth is like our mother; it is where we are born. It is where everything that we have ever experienced has occurred. Unless you are an astronaut, you have only ever been on this earth. You can put your feet in the dirt or sand to feel more connected. You can be surrounded by plants and trees· that fill you with healthy air. Your friends and family that can make you feel better about yourself or a situation. You can be engulfed with love and passion and happiness. All of these things are going to be incredibly important for you.

Not only are you connected to the earth, but you are also connected to your body. Look at all the other animals that surround you. They have bodies too. All bodies are different. Some are big, some are small, some are tall, some are short. Some are healthy, some aren't.

Your body is yours, and it is the only one that you will ever have. We don't know what will happen in this next life and if we get a new body or not. Maybe our body transforms or maybe it just goes away forever, none of this matter now.

Heal yourself, feel your spirit become cleaner, knowing how deeply connected you are to your body. You feel incredibly powerful, safe, and secure. Let go of everything that has happened to you. This is how we can heal our minds. Our minds carry all of our emotional states, they keep around memories that might hurt us, or they make us think darker thoughts that can be challenging to deal with. Your mind is incredibly important as well. We need to clean up this mind. Let all of your thoughts drift away. Think of them like passing raindrops on a car window. They hit the window but then they fall away and dissolve into other little droplets. Let your thoughts heal just like this. You can keep those thoughts around but transform them and learn how to use them. Pull the good and focus on that rather than getting stuck with the negative ones. When you can heal your mind and your body, you are cleansing your soul. You are dedicated to healing. You make it your focus to be as passionate and calm as possible.

Now you are going to become more and more relaxed. This is how you are going to continue to heal.

Spiritual cleansing will always be important for you to feel better. In the end, let your mind drift away, and allow your body to become relaxed and happy. You are clean. You are pure, you are fresh, you are energized, you are rejuvenated. This is all incredibly important and gives us the spiritual healing that we need.

Breathe in for one, two, three, four, and five, and out for five, four, three, two, one. As we count down from twenty, you will either drift off into sleep or move on to a new meditation.

20, 19, 18, 17, 16, 15, 14, 13, 12, 11, 10, 9, 8, 7, 6, 5, 4, 3, 2, 1

CHAPTER 6

Tips for a Deeper Sleep and a Better Lifestyle

TIPS FOR MEDITATION

We will share some more suggestions and tips to allow you to continue with your meditation practice. These are not aimed at making you an expert but just to assist you on the journey. It is not necessary to try all of these tips at the same time. You can try one or two at a time to see if they help you. There will be some that work better than others. Find what's right for you.

Begin Your Practice with 2-Minute Sessions

It may sound like it's pointless to meditate for just two minutes but trust us when we say it's anything but. It's simple to do this and is the easiest way for a beginner to learn to practice meditation. Just dedicate two minutes of each day to meditation. Continue this for a week. It's easier to follow through with these two minutes than pressuring yourself to sit still for half an hour. Once you get used to these two minutes, you can add more minutes the next week and so on. You will soon see that you easily meditate at least 15 minutes daily after a couple of weeks, and that will be more than enough time for most. So don't worry and don't make excuses about not having time. Everyone has two minutes to meditate.

Practice Your Meditation Every Morning

A lot of people say that they will meditate every day in the beginning, but most of them fail to follow through with this claim. Don't assume that you will always remember or be inclined to do it. Commit yourself to meditating every single morning after you wake up. After you wash up, just set aside a few minutes for this and you will see how much better your day goes. Early mornings are considered the best time to meditate.

Don't Worry About the Process and Focus on Beginning the Practice

When people start meditating or think about starting it, they often waste a lot of time and energy worrying about how they should go about it. They waste time in looking up too many methods, finding the perfect mat to sit on, learning chants, etc. All of these are a part of the practice but not the essence of it. You need not spend so much time on this and should try to go with the flow. Just find a comfortable place to sit where you won't be disturbed or distracted by anything. Sitting right on the ground is completely fine and so is sitting on a chair. To begin with, focus less on all this and more on spending two whole minutes just meditating. The stress of these trivial things will hinder your meditation. So, try to get more used to meditating itself and worry about all this later.

Pay Attention to How You Feel

Once you begin meditating, you need to try being more attuned to your personal feelings. Pay attention to how you feel and how this practice is affecting your body. Tune in to the thoughts that pass through your mind. Don't focus on them but notice them as they flow past. Be accepting of all the feelings and thoughts that you experience during meditation. Nothing is wrong or right; so, don't judge yourself for any of it.

Count as Your Breath

Breathing is an important aspect of meditation. Find the right place to meditate and then close your eyes as you sit comfortably. Start concentrating solely on your breathing. Focus on your breath as you inhale and exhale. Notice how you take in air through your nose and into your lungs. Pay attention as it leaves your body. When you take in a breath, count to one. Count two when you breathe out. Continue the counting as you keep breathing and focus on this alone. It will help you focus more.

It Is Okay for Your Thoughts to Wander

The human mind tends to wander a lot, and you need to be more accepting of it as you meditate. You don't have to assume that you are not allowed to think anything when you meditate. This can be impossible to avoid, at least at first. When you meditate, try not to think but be accepting when thoughts come in. When you notice your concentration wandering off from your meditation to your thoughts, push back your mind slowly. It can be disappointing, and you might feel like you are doing it wrong, but it is all right. Just slowly come back when your mind wanders away.

Be More Accepting

Like we already said, it is natural for thoughts to appear as you meditate. Don't be defensive and try to push them away all the time. Instead, be more accepting and allow them to come and pass. Take note of these thoughts, and you can focus on them later. But as you meditate, allow them to come and go naturally. Your thoughts are a part of you, and you need to accept and forgive yourself for everything that you are.

Don't Stress About the Method of Meditation

You might be worried that you are meditating the wrong way at first. A lot of people get stressed about this and think it will be ineffective if they don't practice the right method or do it the right way. The truth is, there is no perfect method of meditation. You can try the various methods we have mentioned and use them as guidelines, but ultimately, you need to do what feels best for you.

Your Mind Doesn't Have to be Empty While Meditating

Some people think that meditation means getting rid of all thoughts and clearing the mind completely. However, this is not true and can be almost impossible for most people. It can be possible to clear your mind out sometimes, but for the most part, it's not what is essential for meditation. It's normal to have thoughts, and you don't have to force yourself to push them all out. Just be more accepting of them and let them pass without focusing on them. Work more on your concentration, and you will see that it gets easier to reduce distracting thoughts over time.

Take Some Time to Accept Your Thoughts and Feelings

As we mentioned repeatedly, having thoughts while meditating is totally normal. When a thought passes through your mind, it is okay to take a moment and pay attention to it. In the beginning, we recommend just letting the thoughts pass and focus more on breathing. But over time, you can try noticing more of your thoughts too. You should avoid focusing on anything negative and try to bring in more positive thoughts. When you notice your thoughts, you will be able to learn more about yourself. But only allow yourself a moment for this before continuing with your meditation.

Learn a Little More about Yourself Every Day

Meditation is not just about improving your focus or being better able to concentrate. It is about helping your mind develop too. When you become more accepting of your thoughts and feelings, you will learn a lot about yourself. Don't push yourself too hard to think or feel a certain way. Be accepting and learn about yourself. No one can know you better than yourself.

Be Your Own Friend

You need to try learning more about yourself, but this should not be done with a mindset of self-analysis and judgment. Instead, be kinder to yourself. Think of it like learning more about someone you like. Accept who you are and be your friend. Don't be cruel and judgmental towards yourself.

Pay Attention to Your Body

After you get better at counting breaths and meditating, you can try something else. Now you should try focusing on your body. Do this with one body part at a time. As you meditate, focus on a specific body part and try to pay attention to how it feels. Start with the lowest point in your body and move on until every part of your body has been acknowledged. This will allow you to pay attention to your body and learn more about it. You will be able to notice if something feels wrong too.

Be Truly Determined

You cannot say you will meditate regularly and then fail to follow through. It is important to dedicate yourself to this practice. Don't take it lightly. Make sure you stick to this resolution for at least a few weeks. Motivate yourself to follow through with it every day. It will soon become a habit, but not if you lack determination right from the beginning.

Meditate, Regardless of Where You Are

It doesn't matter if you're on a trip or have to work overtime on some days. Don't skip your meditation practice. You might reduce the amount of time you can dedicate to it, but you should still meditate. You don't necessarily need that meditation corner in your home for this. It can be done while sitting in a car or even while you sit in your office chair.

Use Guided Meditations

It may seem hard to meditate when you first begin. Guided meditations can be instrumental in this case. Use these audio or video files to help you get started. They are very simple and accommodating regardless of whether you are a beginner or have practiced for some time.

Have Someone to Be Accountable To

If you keep your resolution to meditate to yourself, you are less likely to follow through with it. It will be easy to give up because there is no one to berate you over it. This is why you need to have someone that will hold you accountable. It could be a friend or family member. Just keep checking in with them, and they will help you stay on track. You can also find someone to practice it regularly. This could be someone you live with, work with, or even someone who will go to lessons with you. Finding a network of people who are interested in meditation will help in reinforcing your new good habit. These people can help support you through your journey. You can find online forums or communities of people who practice meditation too.

RELAXING VISUALIZATION

As we go about our daily lives, sometimes our bodies begin to hold onto our tension. The stresses of work, school, or family life can wear anyone down after a while. We deal with the same problems, day after day. What if there was a meditative solution?

Visualization has also been used as a tool to communicate with the universe. Some believe that stating your intention or your desires within your mind is enough to see those goals begin to materialize. It is said that we are spiritual and vibrational creatures with the ability to authorize our own destiny. Today we are going to try a visualization meditation that you can use again and again.

Find a room in which you feel comfortable and safe. Ensure that you will not be disturbed during the course of the meditation. Distractions must be set aside for just a little while, as you venture into your own mind.

Allow your body to seek out a comfortable position. You could lay down or you could sit with your legs cross and your hands resting in your lap. Find where your limbs want to rest before we begin.

When you are relaxed, close your eyes if you are able. Focus only on your breathing and these words. Feel the air filling your belly and your lungs. Feel it leaving your body again and rejoining the air.

If you have a difficult time maintaining this focus, try the following controlled breathing technique. Take a deep breath into the count of three, through your nose. Hold it inside your diaphragm for a count of four. Release the air through your mouth, to another count of three. You can repeat this as many times as you need.

We will begin by relaxing the muscles in your body. Draw your attention to your toes. Become aware of their presence. Let all of the tension drain from them as you continue to relax.

Focus your mind on your feet. Feel the sensations that your body wishes to communicate with you during this time. The tension that you've been holding in the soles of your feet should slowly melt away.

Become aware of your shins and calf muscles. They have worked so hard to move you around today and every day. Listen to this part of your body for a moment before releasing all of the stress that you've been storing. Your body is becoming heavier and heavier as you allow yourself to surrender to relaxation.

Bring your attention to your knees, doing the same thing. Feel the sensations that your body is begging you to notice and then allow the tension to dissipate. Continue listening to the sounds of your breath as you invite calmness into your being.

Feel your thighs. These muscles are used so much in our everyday lives. They help us sit and stand and move. Allow all of the tightness to slowly drift from your body as you move to your pelvis.

The muscles are releasing their tension. You can feel the surface beneath you as it conforms to your body, supporting you. Bring your awareness to your stomach and lower back.

Your muscles and internal organs began to unwind. Your physical being has been doing its best to keep you safe and to fulfill your desires. All of that tension is how returning to the universe.

Bring your mind to your chest, similarly, allowing yourself to let go of the tension. Take a moment to exhale deeply. As you breathe out, so goes all of the tightness from your heart-space and the surrounding area.

Focus your attention on your hands. Your fingers have been moving all day. One-by-one feel the tension as it flows out of your digits. Do the same with your palms and then your wrists.

Feel the sensations in your forearms and then allow the stress and tightness from your day to just float away from your body. You are completely safe and secure at this moment. You are free to place yourself at ease completely.

Bring your thoughts to your biceps and then your shoulders. Allow these muscles to release their tension. You feel as though you are melting into the surface below you. Continue to breathe deeply.

Focus on your neck. Let go of the tightness that you feel within these muscles and then do the same with the back of your head. All of your rigidity is softening as you listen to the sounds of your body. Feel the air exiting your nostrils.

Pay close attention to the muscles of your face. We often furrow our brow and tense our forehead without even realizing it. Let go of this tightness, completely surrender yourself to the moment.

Feel a wash of serenity beginning at the very top of your head. Imagine the warmth as the sensation travels down through your body. It is ridding you of any leftover strain. You feel completely relaxed.

Imagine that you are sitting in a large field outside. You are comfortable and at ease. You are the only person around for miles. It is evening and the sky is darkening.

You sit before a large movie screen that has been set up just for you. There is a projector located behind you and you can hear the mechanical whirring as it's turned on.

The first scene that you will see on this screen is one that explains your current state of being. The part of your life that you wish to change is what we will focus on. If you are looking for love, then see yourself alone. If you wish to heal an injury, then see that injury occurring.

Do not spare yourself from feeling the pain associated with your current situation. You want to see and feel everything, even though it is negative. We are doing this for a reason. You are reminding yourself of everything that you wish to change. Feeling your dismay for the way things are is going to fuel your metamorphosis. Dwell in your suffering for a moment.

Imagine that you are standing up and turning the projector off. This is a gesture that communicates that you have control over the situation. You are choosing to change your own life.

I want you to think of a goal, something that you wish to achieve. This can be anything from a vacation you want to go on to a promotion at your job. There is no dream too large or small. Imagine what life would look like if you achieved this particular goal.

See yourself on the giant screen before you. It is a snapshot of your life after your goal has been achieved. You must immerse yourself in this experience. Do your best to feel the sensations and emotions. Pay attention to the look on your face and on the faces of those around you. Hear the sounds that you would hear in that situation. What do you smell? Taste? It is also known to be helpful if you see at least two other people in your scene, who are positively impacted by the achievement of your goals.

Watch the scene before you unfold. See the colors becoming more and more vivid than they were before. It is as though you are making this image slowly come to life. You are at that moment. You are watching a reality where you have made your dreams come true. Feel all of the good emotions associated with your success.

Now watch as the screen displays your life a year after your goal has been achieved. Pay attention again, to the sensations, sounds, and smells. You want to see the screen in vivid color. Spend as much time as you need here.

When you have finished with your meditations, spend a few moments in quiet contemplation before you rejoin the world. Do this exercise a few times a week. Use this time to communicate with yourself and with the world outside you. This meditation is a statement of your intentions to the universe.

POSITIVE AFFIRMATIONS FOR BETTER SLEEP

An affirmation is an affirming statement that you make to yourself in order to reiterate the importance of an idea. Throughout the day, you might think of negative affirmations that validate your perspective. These can include things like, "I'm not good enough," or "Nothing is going right in my life." These statements aren't necessarily the whole truth, but they might have a certain element that can help solidify one perspective.

These affirmations are going to help you focus on what's most important and remember the ideas needed in order to get your best night's sleep possible. Repeat these back to yourself, write them down and make notes around your home, or simply remember them in your mind when you need them the most.

Affirmations for Failing and Staying Asleep

The best way to include these affirmations in your life is to repeat them daily. They will help retrain your brain to think more positively rather than the negative ways that you might be thinking now.

In order to reiterate the importance of affirmations, including physical activity can help you to remember them even more. When you integrate a physical exercise with a mental thought, it helps make it more real. It will be easier to accept these affirmations in your life when an emphasis is put on truly believing them.

The first movement that you can do in order to remember these exercises is to hold an item physically.

As you are saying these affirmations, physically touch and hold these items. Let it remind you of reality. Stay focused and grounded on remembering the most important aspects of these affirmations.

Alternatively, try implementing new breathing exercises that we haven't tried yet. The method of breathing in through your nose and out through your mouth is important, but as we go further, there are other ways that you can include healthy breathing with these positive sleep affirmations.

One method is breathing through alternate nostrils. Make a fist with your right hand with your thumb and pinky sticking out. Take your pinky and place it on your left nostril, closing it so that you can only breathe through one.

Now, breathing for five counts through that nostril.

Then, take your right thumb, and place it on your right nostril, closing that and releasing your pinky from the other nostril. Now, breathe out for five.

You will notice that doing this breathing exercise on its own is enough to help you be more relaxed. Now, when you pair it with the affirmation that we're about to read aloud, you will start to put more of an emphasis on creating thinking patterns around these affirmations.

An alternate method of breathing is to breathe in for three counts, say the affirmation, and then breathe out for three counts. You can do this on your own with the affirmations that are most important to your life.

It will be beneficial for you to have a journal that you keep affirmations in as well. Have one hand to write these affirmations down as they apply to your life. Writing about them will help you remember them and keep a note of the things that are most effective in your life.

When you are having a bad day, you can visit these affirmations. When you need a little confidence booster, or some motivation, use these affirmations.

We will now get into the reading of these. Remember to focus on your breathing as we take you through these, and if you are not planning on drifting off to sleep once they have finished, taking notes can help as well.

Healthy Sleep Dedication

I am dedicated to making healthy choices for my sleeping habits.

The things that I do throughout my day will affect how I sleep; therefore, I am going to make sure to focus on making the best choices for all aspects of my health.

I will do things that aren't always easy because it will be in the best interest of my health overall.

When I am well-rested, everything else in my life becomes easier.

I am more focused when I have slept an entire night, so I know that falling asleep is incredibly important to my health.

Developing healthy habits is easy when I dedicate my time towards a better future.

It feels good to take care of myself.

I deserve a good night's sleep; therefore, I deserve everything else that will come along with this benefit.

I am naturally supposed to get rest. It is not wrong for me to be tired and to choose to do healthy things for my sleep cycles.

Dreams are normal, and I am focused on embracing them and avoiding nightmares.

I choose to go to bed at a decent time at night because it is best for my health.

Whatever is waiting for me tomorrow will still be there whether I get a full night's sleep or not, so it is best to ensure I am getting the proper amount of rest.

I take care of my body because I know that it is the only one that I will ever have.

I allow discipline in my life to guide me in the right direction to make the choices that are healthiest for my individual and specific lifestyle.

I nourish my body and make sure I get the right amount of nutrients to keep me energized throughout the day.

I am strong because I get the right amount of sleep.

Getting the right kind of sleep is good for my mental health.

I am happier when I am well-rested. I am in a better mood and can laugh more easily when I have had a good night's sleep.

I am grateful for my opportunity to be healthier and to get better sleep.

I am thankful that I have the ability to make the right choices for my health and overall wellbeing.

Having habits is not a bad thing; I just need to make sure that my habits are healthy ones.

I am less stressed out when I am able to get a better night's sleep.

I am the best version of myself when I am healthy. I am healthiest when I am well-rested and focused on getting a better night's sleep.

Everything else in my life will fall into place as I focus on getting the best night's sleep possible.

I love myself; therefore, I am going to put an emphasis on dedication to better sleeping habits so that I can feel better all the time.

Relaxing

I am feeling relaxed.

Relaxation is a feeling I can elicit, not a state that I have to be in depending

on certain restrictions.

I can feel the relaxation in my mind first and foremost.

As I feel my body becoming relaxed, I can feel that serenity pass through the upper half of my body.

All of the tension that I might have built throughout the day is now starting to fade away.

I am focused on myself and centered within my body.

I can tell that my muscles are becoming more and more relaxed. There is nothing that concerns me at the moment.

There will always be stressors in my life, but right now, I do not have to worry about any of those.

As I focus on being calmer, it is easier for my mind to relax. I do not have to be afraid of what happened in the past.

I cannot change the things that are already written in history. I don't need to be fearful of the future.

I can make assumptions, but my predictions will not always be accurate. I can focus on the now, which is the most important thing to do.

As I start to draw my attention to the present moment, I find it easier to relax.

The more relaxed I am, the easier it will be for me to fall asleep. The faster I fall asleep, the more rest that I can get.

I have no concern over what is going on around me. The only thing I am concerned with is being relaxed in the present moment.

I exude relaxation and peace. Others will notice how quiet, calm, and collected I can be.

I am balanced in my stress and pleasure aspects, meaning that I have less anxiety.

I am not afraid of being stressed.

Stress helps me remember what is most important in my life. Stress keeps me focused on my goals.

I do not let this stress consume me.

I manage my stress in healthy and productive ways.

I have the main control over the stress that I feel. No one else is in charge of my feelings.

It is normal for me to be peaceful.

I allow this lifestyle to take over every aspect, making it easier to have a more relaxed sleep.

When I can truly calm myself down all the way, it will be easier to stay asleep.

I let go of my anxiety because it serves me no purpose. I am excited for the future.

I am not afraid of any of the challenges that I might face. It is easy for me to be more and more relaxed.

There is nothing more freeing than realizing that I do not have to be anxious over certain aspects in my life.

I will sleep easier and more peacefully knowing that there is nothing in this world that I need to be afraid of.

Staying Asleep

Nothing feels better than crawling into my bed after a long day.

My bedroom is filled with peace and serenity. I have no trouble drifting off to sleep.

Everything in my room helps me to be more relaxed.

I feel safe and at peace knowing that I am protected in my room.

I have no trouble falling asleep once I am able to close my eyes and focus on my breathing.

I make sure all of my anxieties are gone so that I can fall asleep easier.

When bad thoughts come into my head, I know how to push them away so that I can focus instead on getting a better night's sleep.

I am centered on reality, which involves getting the best sleep possible. It is so refreshing to wake up after a night of rest that was uninterrupted.

Any time that I might wake up, I have no trouble knowing how to get myself back to sleep.

Whenever I wake up, it is easy to get out of bed within the first few times that my alarm clock rings.

The better night's sleep I get, the easier it is for me to wake up. I release all of the times that I have had a restless night's sleep.

No matter how many times I have snuggled with my sleep in the past, I know that I am capable of getting the best night's sleep possible.

HOW TO FORM GOOD HABITS

To form good habits, you need to make a conscious and deliberate effort on your part to achieve it. Good habits are easy to form if you have the discipline to do so.

It is easy to hear your friend, or a colleague say he wants to do this or that and he gets it done and when you try to do the same it doesn't work out. Forming a good habit can be a struggle at times but if you are determined and patient, it can change. However, forming a good habit takes time for you to become glued to it.

Consistency

The world consistency implies that you are ready to make sacrifices to enable you to sustain your habits. Consistency is the essential requirement you need to form good habits. Consistency will make you stop seeing your pattern as chores. Consistency will help follow your set goals. In all honesty, you can't form good habits without consistency.

Make Plans and Set Goals

Making plans and have set goals of the habits you want to form is the first step towards forming a good habit. Making a plan and setting goals implies that you take a critical look at what you hope to gain from the intended habit. Is the habit worth it? Is it achievable? Is it even realistic? All these questions are what you will be able to answer after you make plans and set goals about the good habit you want to form.

For example, you want to form the habit of exercising regularly. During the process of making plans and setting goals, you will know why you want to start exercising regularly, how you can achieve success when you should start as well as what you should gain from it. Like I stated earlier, making plans, and set goals are essential to forming a good habit.

Have a Little Beginning

Often when you hear people complaining that they find it difficult to form good habits or do good things regularly, it has to do with them trying to go the full 9- yards too soon. If you look at people who want to lose weight, for example, and trying to make fitness a habit, you will discover one thing most of the do. They ignore starting small. They want to do 1km walk in a week; they want to do 100 push-ups in 2 days. While it is good to start, it often requires a tremendous amount of will power to archive this level of hard work. Most beginners do have the required willpower to pull it off, and that makes the habit fail.

However, if you start small, let's say rather than 1km walk, do a 100m or a 50. Instead of 100 push-ups, start with a 20 and work your way up. Starting small will make you not see your newly formed habit as a chore that needs to be done but rather as a way to relax and have fun. Starting small will reduce the amount of willpower you will need to accomplish to sustain your habit.

Recognize the Importance of Time

Forming a new habit requires a significant amount of time. Don't expect to start something in a day, and it will become a habit the next. Things don't work that way. Recognize the vitality of time and give yourself some. You are allowed to do that. Giving yourself a little time to make your habit automatic will help you overcome frustration - which is one of the things that can destroy the habit you are trying to form.

Know Your Motivation

Ordinarily, this should be part of setting goals I spoke about earlier, but I feel the need to explain it in more detail. Having the right motivation can go a long way to ensure you maintain your habit for as long as possible. The right motivation will give you a boost when you no longer feel you can continue with your good habit.

For example, if you wish to form the habit of losing weight, writing your source of motivation down will give you a boost when you feel like you can't go on.

Change Your Thinking (Become More Mindful)

Lots of individuals are on autopilot nowadays. The autopilot behavior makes it hard for them to form new good habits. The reason is they are not thinking of what they are doing or ought to do. However, to form new good habits, become more mindful of your actions. Becoming more conscious of what you are doing will help you keep better track of time and help you maintain your newly formed good habits.

Furthermore, a change of mindset is essential to form good habits. The reason is the mind controls the body. For you to conquer your old ways and form a new good one, you need to overcome the old one in your mind first. A change in mindset will bring a change in behavior and also give you a boost.

Associate with Supporters

Your friends and family can help you form a good habit and help you break old ones as well. The support of friends will serve as motivation to maintain your newly formed good habits.

For example, if you want to form the habit of eating healthy, you need to be friends who share a similar lifestyle, or it will be difficult for you to follow through with your new good habit.

In a nutshell, if you have friends who don't share the same habit with you or don't want even to try, it is time to make new friends.

Alter Your Environment

The environment we find ourselves in plays a vital role in our growth, character, and habits as well. For an individual who is in an environment where lots of people are obese and don't eat healthily, it will be difficult for that person to form a habit of eating healthy. Therefore, if you want to form a habit of eating healthy, it is time to make a change. Move to a different environment or try to make the people around you join you in your new habit.

The same thing applies to a person who wants to form the habit of going to the gym every day. You can work or change your environment by having your gym bag at the side of your bed at night. You can also lay your gym clothes on your bed or hang them at the door of your bathroom. So, you can see it before you enter to have a shower in the morning.

Involve People

To maintain your new habit, and focus on your goals, get people involved. Tell people about the new habit you want to form. These people will help you stay in-line when you begin to lose sight of what you're doing. These people will hold you accountable for your newly formed habit. They will make you stay committed to the course.

For you to get people to help you focus, try to have a sort of way, your friend will hold you accountable. You can give out your property or some money to them and tell them to hold it until you have committed to your habit completely.

Personalize and Celebrate Your Victory

Often times, we berate ourselves for not doing the right thing. However, we should learn to give ourselves credit when we do the right thing as well.

When you want to form a new good habit, it is good for you to celebrate your success in meeting your goals for the day.

As you commit to your newly formed habit, celebrating your success by rewarding yourself for committing to your new habit will help you stay motivated. Motivation is vital when trying to create a new good pattern. For example, if your new habit is to lose weight, you can reward yourself with new cloth whenever you lose a couple of pounds. If your new habit is to eat healthily, you can reward yourself by taking yourself out to dinner once a week or so for maintaining your healthy lifestyle. Doing this all the time will motivate you.

Create a Cue Around Your Habit

When trying to form a new good habit, it is to find yourself lacking the motivation and courage to go through with your habit. Imagine a scenario when your alarm goes off at 6:30 am. Immediately you get up, your first thought will be to have your bath and get ready for work. But if your habit is on cue, for example, you have a friend to meet at the gym at 7:30 am, and you wouldn't want to disappoint him. So, you will force yourself to go to the gym that morning. Another thing you can do is to talk about your newly formed good habit on social media like Facebook.

Talking about your new habit on social will make you stay committed to it as you would not like to let your friends down.

Form a pattern with your Habit

Forming a pattern gets a lot of things done. I once had a friend who was able to write five articles a day because he was able to form a pattern around his writing. He wrote his articles before having breakfast. He kept to the pattern for 30 days straight. By the time he noticed how much work he gets done in a day, he had already established a pattern; he didn't want to break.

You can factor this into your newly formed good habit as well. Set your new good habit to form a pattern, and you will be able to sustain it.

Expect Setbacks

The simple fact is nothing good comes easy. This is a known fact. Farming a new good habit is no different. You should expect setbacks as you try to form a new good habit. You must expect this setback because it will help you overcome them. It is good for you to have at the back of your mind that stumbling along the way doesn't mean you can't continue working to form a new habit. Setbacks are to serve as motivation and not to discourage you.

For instance, if you fail to make it to your gym appointment, don't get discouraged. Reschedule your date and try to make it this time.

CHAPTER 7

Bedtime Stories to Relieve Anxiety and Fall Asleep

SHORT STORIES AGAINST ANXIETY AND STRESS TO HELP ADULT FALL ASLEEP

Denmark is high up north, where Germany stops. There is still a king there today, but he is no longer there to govern, but usually visits kindergartens because his wife likes children so much.

But a long time ago, the Danish king was very powerful. As all kings used to do, he always wanted to increase his land so that he would become even more powerful. So, he also had to conquer another country. That was not easy. In the south of Denmark was Germany, then the kingdoms of Hanover and Prussia. He could not mess with them because they had many more soldiers than him. Likewise, the Swedes, whose country lies next to Denmark.

So, he looked north. Far behind the sea was Greenland. This is a huge country, but at the time it was very little known, and it was supposed to be very cold there. So, he had three ships loaded from the royal fleet. On each he put a brave knight and several soldiers, as well as horses and all kinds of war equipment.

Then it went off to Greenland in the terribly cold north. When the ships arrived, they first saw a lot of ice and snow. The knights put on their armor and went ashore to conquer it. But no one was visible, and the knights froze in their iron armor on the ice, so they could not move. They kicked wildly, clawing their iron armor hard to free themselves from the ice.

A few of the other soldiers had to make a fire to get them released. As a result, of course, the armor on the feet were pretty hot and the knights burned their feet. They shopped around wildly until they were finally free and quickly disappeared on the ship.

Then one tried to bring the horses ashore, because one should conquer Greenland. The horses struggled hard, but after a few meters they also got stuck in the snow. The soldiers could not walk in the high snow and froze miserably, so that finally all went with their horses back on the ships and Greenland could not conquer first. When the knights sat around thinking and pondering, the lookout on the ship's mast reported "Enemy ahead!!"

And indeed, the knights saw in astonishment how a sleigh came with very small horses. They were astonished even more when they discovered that it was not horses but many dogs in front of a sled so effortlessly whizzing across the snow.

Everyone brought their rifles and lances and feared that they would have to defend themselves. But there was only one man on the sled, an Eskimo. He greeted them in a very friendly way and was happy to see so many people, because in Greenland not so many people live, and one is often quite lonely and alone. He welcomed everyone and asked them if they would not visit him in the evening, his wife would cook a nice soup of seal meat for them.

From whom you are greeted so friendly, you can fight badly against, and so put three of the knights on the dogsled, but without their heavy armor. Husch - you rushed over the landscape to a strange hut, which was made entirely of snow. It's called an igloo and its round, but it's very nice and warm!

When they had eaten, they thanked each other, and the Eskimo drove them back to their ships by dog sled. Then it was decided to drive back to Denmark.

They then reported everything to the king. He held advice with his ministers on how to conquer Greenland. They also asked a wise older man named Count Johannsen. The count whispered his suggestion in the ear of the king, and he was thrilled!

He sent his steward to the city to buy whatever vanilla powder he could get. Then he equipped a ship again, but this time the knights should put on thick fur coats and take sledges with them. In addition, the whole load compartment was full of vanilla powder!

Arrived in Greenland, they were greeted by Eskimos again, it was already known by now. The soldiers from Denmark brought a lot of fresh snow and made it with their vanilla powder from delicious vanilla ice cream. They gave it to the Eskimos.

They had never eaten anything like that! They were crazy about it and still wanted to have more. The knights, however, kept everything under wraps and first wanted to speak to the eskimo leader, who was quickly brought for them. With him, the knights made a contract that now Greenland would belong to Denmark and for that the Eskimos would get as much vanilla ice cream as they could eat.

Then the knights sailed home with their ship and told their king that Greenland would now belong to Denmark, without there being a war! And that's how it is today so that you can ask every Dane.

FALLING ASLEEP IN A RAINFOREST-BEDTIME STORY

As you listen to me and begin to fall asleep, I'm going to tell you a story in the background. And as you drift comfortably asleep, you can have a sense of somebody who was going about everyday life, waking up, going through their life, going to work, being polite to others, going home, watching some TV going to bed, getting up, going to work, being polite to others, going home and watching some TV and going to bed. And every day this was their routine. They would wake up, go to work, go home, watch TV and go to bed. Then one day, they woke up and they thought to themselves that they didn't want to keep doing this. They wished that there was something more exciting in life, because when they were thinking back over their past, only a few memories stood out. Most of the memories just blurred into one. They couldn't tell one day from the next, just getting up, going to work, going home, watching TV and going to bed.

One day while they were at home, they decided to take a look on the internet and randomly book a holiday. A trip anywhere at all, they didn't know where, they just wanted to book something. They booked a holiday to an exotic location and all of a sudden while they were going to work, they found themselves thinking about the excitement of the trip away that they had coming up in the future. While they were at work working and smiling politely, they were, in their minds, thinking about what this exotic location would be like. On their journey home they were thinking about that holiday they were going to be going on and looking forward to it. And every day they crossed off a date on the diary as they got closer and closer to their trip. And then the holiday came around and they travelled to that exotic location, the plane landed, they went to the hotel and left their stuff in the hotel. They decided to go out exploring. They went out exploring and wandered out into a beautiful rainforest. Listening to the sounds of the birds, the rustling of the leaves, the sounds of monkeys in the distance and all of the other sounds.

They could feel how warm it was in the rainforest. Their attention was so focused on the excitement on the exploration. They could hear water in the distance and so they pushed through the rainforest. The sound of the water got louder and louder and they continued pushing through the rainforest excitedly, wondering what they would find. The sound of the water continued to get louder and louder until eventually they found a clearing. Suddenly there was the light from the sun beating down on them, that glistened on the water of the giant lake surrounded by huge waterfalls. They could see huge waterfalls and the spray and mist coming up from the bottom of the waterfalls and rainbows dancing in the spray above the lake. They saw what looked like a small wooden boat down on the lake, they walked down to the boat, climbed into the boat, picked up the oars, pushed off the side and gently paddled out into the lake. They could feel the force of the water against the oars as they paddled. They paddled out towards the center of the lake. The lake was calm here in the center, the water quickly calming as it moved away from the waterfalls. The lake appeared to be deep. The person pulled the oars into the boat, put their backpack down to use as a pillow, laid back in the boat, closed their eyes and relaxed listening to the waterfalls in the background, smelling the freshwater air. Feeling the subtlest rocking of the boat on the lake and feeling the warmth of the sun beating down on them.

With their eyes closed, they took some deep breaths and relaxed. They allowed themselves to become absorbed in the moment. And as they relaxed and became absorbed in the moment, the sun continued its journey across the sky, gradually lowering in the sky and the sounds in the forest began to change, from daytime sounds to nighttime sounds. And as the sun set, the person opened their eyes and gazed up into the sky. And as they gazed up into the sky, they could see the blanket of stars twinkling, different colors in the sky, different clouds. And they could see the Milky Way stretching across the sky. They recognized one point of light in the sky as being Mars. And as they gazed at that point of light, as they gazed up at Mars, their eyes began to close again. And as their eyes began to close, they discovered their eyes opening actually on the red planet. And oddly they didn't have any space gear on, and they were able to breathe perfectly fine, as if they were just on Earth, but they know they were on the red planet.

And they discovered themselves at the foot of a mountain range on Mars. And they thought "Wouldn't it be exciting to climb a mountain range on Mars?" And so, they climbed the mountain, they trekked up the mountain. And as they approached the summit, they noticed how vibrant the color red was. They began to get a new perspective on this world. They sat down and they enjoyed the view, knowing they were the first person ever to step foot here. And as the small sun set on Mars, they could see two small moons in the sky and all of the stars in the sky and they could see off in the distance, a pale blue dot and they knew it was Earth. And they enjoyed the awe, the wonder of gazing at that pale blue dot. Knowing all life on Earth, all known life in the universe, is on that pale blue dot. Suddenly they had a sense that life seems so fragile when it is all contained in that one location and such a small location from this distance. They felt a sense of love and compassion for all that life. And a sense of the importance of looking after that pale blue dot. And as the sun rose on another Martian day, with these new learnings they climbed down the mountain. And as they reached the base of the mountain, they found their eyes opening in the boat floating on the lake, listening to that water, feeling the warmth of the morning sun.

They got the oars and rowed back to shore. They continued exploring for a while in the rainforest before deciding to pitch up a tent to camp in the rainforest. They pitched the tent up tied between the trees, positioned a few feet off the ground where you can climb up into the tent and be a few feet off the ground. In the tent, you feel like you are floating. And as they relaxed in the tent, feeling comfortable and calm, so they noticed how their tent sways gently between the trees, almost like being rocked gently to sleep and they did, rock gently to sleep in the tent. And after a week or so, of enjoying this exotic holiday seeing colorful birds, seeing different apes and other animals, taking plenty of photographs and writing down thoughts that came to mind. Then they took down their tents and travelled back home and they appreciated their own bed more than they had appreciated it in a long time. And they knew they had to do this more often as they relaxed down in their bed and drifted comfortably and deeply asleep.

MOTHER'S LOVE BEDTIME STORY

On a summer's day, a little boy walked through a flower field.

He saw beautiful flowers and wanted to pick them for his dear mother.

What the boy did not know was that his father, who lived in the underworld, had deliberately planted beautiful flowers for the boy so that he could take him to his dark world.

He knew that the innocent, sweet boy did not want to go to his dark underground world.

The boy saw a lovely white rose; he wanted to pick it because he knew that this was a lovely rose. The rose was huge and seemed to radiate a beautiful rainbow-like aura. They looked like prisms. The boy bent over and picked the white rose for his mother. And as he stooped, the earth suddenly split up at his feet, and he just disappeared under the ground.

In the underground world, his father took him on his massive span of black horses.

The boy cried and called for his dear mother, but she could no longer help him there in the underworld. She couldn't even hear him there so far away from her hearing.

But her heart had already heard of it, and she stared in the great silence. Something had happened to her child, but what?

She did not know and went searching quickly.

She searched and searched for hours until dark came, but she could not find her child again.

Tired of crying and shouting, she went back to the house, where an old owl was sitting in the tree next to their home.

Oh, owl tells me, do you know where my son is? I lost him, she exclaimed desperately.

Owl said to the owl, and after this, he replied: Your child has been seen at the bottom of the earth, with his father he will be and stay how you will get him back.

The mother fell to the ground and ran her fingers into the earth. "Oh, dear son, come back to me", she cried.

But she couldn't reach him in that underground.

In the meantime, the boy also cried in the underground for his mother, there with his father.

It made the father tired and very angry.

Stop crying, mom's baby. Stop it, I tell you. But the boy was inconsolable.

He loved his mother dearly, and even though this was his father, his father lived in the underground and wanted to live in the sun with his mother, not in the dark.

The father brought out all kinds of toys and crayons and paper; he tried to make the child laugh, but nothing helped.

The darkness in the underground became even darker, the atmosphere even grimmer, and nothing brought joy or relief.

The father was the devil.

Once he had fallen in love with the beautiful goddess daughter on earth, he had spied on her, and while he was looking at her, he had fallen madly in love and had taken her to the darkness of his underworld.

She had first cried, and after a while, resigned but accepted that he was holding her captive.

He often brought her flowers and the tastiest snacks. But he couldn't make her happy.

One day she had asked him something that he agreed to because he saw how unhappy she was there with him in that unde1world.

She had asked him if he wanted to release her, but he had told her that he would then have a child of hers, after which she was free to go.

She had not spoken to him for three months, but after that, she had said yes.

Not long after, it turned out that she was blessed with a child. He was pleased but also sad; he had to let her go if she had given birth to their child.

She was also thrilled, but also sad; she had to let her child go if she had given birth to them.

The child was born one day in the summer. He was a beautiful boy, and both parents were thrilled. They loved the child very much. The mother was free to go, yet she couldn't do this yet, she couldn't say goodbye to her child. So, she stayed and stayed longer and longer.

One day, she walked with the child in her arms along an underground brook, with a tall tree beside it with the crown very far away into the earth of the roof.

And suddenly, a ray of sunshine shone through it; the mother then knew how much she had missed the sun and the earth above it.

The child on her arm sneezed in the bright sun on his face and in his clear blue eyes.

The mother laughed at this.

She lovingly kissed the child's nose and came up with a plan.

The next day she returned with a long flight of stairs and escaped with her child towards the earth and the sun. She was so happy!!!

She had escaped that man and still had her child.

After many years the father had sworn revenge; she had left him with their baby.

That would regret her.

That is why the day came when the father came to claim the child.

The mother was desperate with grief. She searched and dug in the earth for an entrance to the underworld but could not find it anymore.

Many animals from the nearby forest came to help the mother and dug burrows to an underworld.

But they too could not get that far.

One day the mother went to a witch. The witch told her that she had to complete three tasks and that she could revisit her child afterward.

The mother agreed; she would do whatever the witch expected of her.

The mother sets off to get 1 golden feather from the king's hen house.

That is not easy because this chicken henhouse consists of all expensive chickens which are protected by 3 large guard dogs.

When the mother arrives at the royal chickens, she softly shouts, Holy Mother Chicken?

Holy mother hen?

Chaos arises; all chickens drift apart and start cackling that it is a sweet delight.

The guard dogs suddenly stand around the mother, with a dangerous growl, they bare their teeth. What are you looking for the boy's mother here, a guard dog asks viciously?

I am looking for my child, so I do what I have to do. Why do you have to do this, the other guard dog snarls?

Because it is my child, therefore, the mother defends her child.

The one watchdog starts to howl. I also have a young one, and he is in pain and can no longer walk.

I will look at it, the mother says kindly, but then I have to get the golden feather from mother chicken in return.

No sooner said than done, the mother heals the paw of the pup of the guard dog, there was a thorn in his paw, and the mother gets the golden feather from mother chicken.

The first assignment was fulfilled; the mother happily goes back to the witch.

The old witch says nicely, looking at the golden feather in her hand, and now the next assignment.

PEACE OF MIND BEDTIME STORY

Frances had been granted the gift of mind-reading from a very young age. It was a completely anomalous occurrence, as no one in her family had the ability, and no one could discern how Frances had come to possess the power. It was simply something she knew how to do, and it was something her parents had to work very hard to get around.

They spent time helping her differentiate between the things that people said with their minds and what they said with their mouths. They helped her to realize that she should not comment on the things they were thinking unless it became absolutely necessary for her to do so.

There were plenty of awkward moments amongst the family when Frances was easily able to discern whether someone had been lying to her, whether it was for her own good or not. Most of the time, her parents did their best to level with her and to keep their thoughts civil while she was around. This was quite an interesting exercise in self-discipline.

As Frances got older, she began to understand boundaries, and she began to become more comfortable with compartmentalizing people so the things they said were kept separate from the things they thought. She didn't want to invade anyone's privacy with her gift, it simply happened to her. She could typically tune it out if the thoughts were benign enough, but she would occasionally hear something that would set her teeth on edge, or which would completely put her off of someone's company.

This gift had made things a little bit more difficult, it seemed, when it came to the subject of meeting someone special. Any time she wanted to engage in a relationship with someone, she would find them thinking repugnant, distracting, or downright confusing things that she didn't know how to look past. She would always find herself grappling with the thoughts her partner was having, rather than being able to relate to them comfortably.

Her mother had tried to walk her through the parts of dating that were not completely foreign to her, but modern dating was different. Modern dating, plus the ability to read someone's mind was even more so. It seemed like no matter what advise her mother gave her, she couldn't seem to get ahead of the curve on what random guys in the dating scene were going to be thinking at any given time.

She went on one date with a man named Jared, who looked like a really nice guy. He had pretty brown eyes, neat brown hair, glasses, and he dressed so nicely for his date with Frances. They talked about the things they were looking for in potential partners and the things that came up were somewhat distracting.

"I think I'm just looking for someone that I can talk to about things without feeling pressure to be on my A-game all the time. Someone who has slip-ups themselves from time to time and someone who can roll with the punches in life," he said to her.

"Yes, I definitely agree with that! I hate feeling like I have to stand on ceremony for people in my life."

Then you'd hate my mother. My mother would probably hate you too, though. Speaking of which, I should call her. Should I go to the bathroom and call her now?

"Yeah! You know, I actually have to go to the bathroom for a minute. I'll be right back."

Jared spent about thirty minutes in that bathroom before Frances decided it was probably best just to call it a night. She paid half of the bill and left.

Christopher had shaggy blonde hair and seemed like he was more the type just to relax and let things roll off his shoulders. They got a beer, sat down, and before anyone could say anything, he had a rather loud thought.

Wow, I can't believe she sat down before me. What a selfish hag.

Frances did her best to push the thought away. Perhaps she had misunderstood.

"So, Christopher, do you have any hobbies or interests?" She scarcely heard what his response really was over the intrusive thought that came next.

Of course, I have hobbies and interests, idiot. What kind of one-dimensional toad do you think I am? Why am I even wasting my time with this witch? She's probably terrible in bed.

Frances looked him squarely in the eyes and said, "You might want to see a therapist about your anger issues." She stood up from the table without another word and walked out of the restaurant. She truly did hope he got the help he needed, but she would not sit there and listen to the vitriol he had to spew in the meantime.

She had all but given up hope of finding someone compatible when a dating app she had downloaded pinged her. Derek wants to connect! It said cheerily. She rolled her eyes, but she decided to check the app anyway. What could it hurt to listen to a few more ridiculous thoughts before giving up completely on the concept of finding love?

She opened the app and saw a very nice smile on a man with dark hair, light blue eyes, and tan skin. His profile said he was interested in hiking, casual get-togethers, bonfires, friends, and music.

Hiking was about the only thing on there that Frances didn't quite identify with, but she could learn to love hiking if it came down to it. She could do with a little more time in the great outdoors, and she could use a little more physical activity. The only reason she never did anything like that, she was reasonably convinced, was because she didn't have anyone to go with.

She messaged Derek and set up a time and place to meet him. She got to the restaurant, and he had already gotten them a table and was waiting for her to arrive. He stood up and greeted her warmly. She was surprised by how instantly welcome she felt when she got to the table.

They introduced themselves and got into casual conversation. She was surprised that they had exchanged pleasantries and she had yet to hear a thought that set her teeth on edge. Or any kind of thought at all.

They talked for a while and he seemed to have real depth to him, in spite of the fact that she couldn't hear thoughts coming from him. She smiled at him for a moment.

"I can't tell what you're thinking," she blurted happily.

"Oh, I know. My friends tell me that I'm a completely closed book. The thing is, I meditate a lot and I've learned how to keep my head clear when I'm talking to people. It's a really valuable skill that keeps me from sticking my foot in my mouth. You'd be shocked how often I would say something completely asinine without even realizing I had done it." She held up her phone and wiggled it.

"I've been meeting guys on this app for a couple of months now; I think I might have some idea of how often guy's brains betray them." He laughed heartily.

Frances found herself thinking that there may yet have been hope to find love.

THE DREAM LIFE BEDTIME STORIES

Just when you think life cannot get any worse than it currently is, either something magical can happen that will change your luck, or it gets a little bit worse. Those are the only two options, after today you wonder how your luck will go, will it be better? Or will your life come crashing down around you? You hear a knock on the door, your tired body drags you to answer it. You open the door to see a businesswoman, smiling largely as she hands you a heavy briefcase. Puzzled you don't want her to release the case. Who is this woman? Why is she here? Your brain struggles to process this, then she starts talking.

"You are the winner of the dream life sweepstake. You are the luckiest person on Earth right now, and everything is going to change for the better." This feels like a gimmick, surely, she will say you only need to invest, blah, blah, blah. So, you tell her that you are not interested, and you just want her to leave you in peace so you can rest. She is dumbfounded as you shut the door in her face.

As you walk back to your bed, your phone rings. You answer it to hear a formal voice on the other line announce that he's a lawyer for the World's richest man, a man who died a few weeks ago. In his will he had a list of names, people that he had encountered in his life...everyone from the school librarian in primary school to a drive thru window cashier at the McDonald's. Anyone he met; he added them to this list. Upon his death he wanted his list to become a sweepstakes for his fortune, but his money ruined his life. It tore apart his family, it made him greedy, it made him lazy. He wants someone to be able to live out their dream life, through his will, but with guidance. The lady at the door is the first step towards guiding you to accepting this fortune. After the lawyer explains, you still can't seem to process this. You don't think you met this man, and if you had...would you be so lucky as to win his entire fortune?

Is this that point where your luck changes? Will it be the best thing that ever happened to you? Or will you waste your time? Isn't it worth the amount of time, just to listen to the lady? What harm can it do? You turn around and walk back to the door. Allowing the woman to enter your home. You have a seat at the table, and she opens the brief case. "First, we will start with a questionnaire. I am to guide you to a dream life, not just hand you a fortune. Once I am certain you are ready to have the fortune, it will be all yours." You hesitantly agree, still feeling this is too good to be true.

What is your dream job, do you wish to earn fulfillment through your work, or is it a means to an end? You decide you have nothing to hide from this woman, so you tell her the truth. She nods and moves on to the next question.

What is your dream family? Do you have it? Would money change your family, for the better or for the worse?

If you could live anywhere in the world, where would you live? Why would you live there?

"Ok, that takes care of the basics. Give me a few moments and I'll be back soon." As she leaves the room, you suddenly find yourself a bundle of nerves. Your body is tense and achy. You want to relax yourself, not let this work you up. So, you take a deep breath in as you stretch and flex the muscles in your body. As you exhale slowly, you allow the muscles to relax. You can feel a warm tingling sensation rushing through as you repeat the process. You keep breathing in slowly, becoming aware of your body. It is heavy and tired, you relax into the chair and focus on the simple task of breathing and allowing your body to rest. The lady enters the room again and you feel relaxed, maybe this is for the best. "Now, we will start building your dream. life. Starting with some major purchases, then working through the minor ones so we can organize your new life. What type of car do you wish to have? Do you need anything custom on it?" She hands you a form, as you order your dream car.

You think about all the cars you've wanted throughout your life, until you finally settle on one. You try to keep it in mind, this is because you're not spending your own money. This is just a 'dream' car for a reason. Think of every elaborate detail you would want in that car, including a personal driver, if that's what you want. Once you have etched every detail into that paper, hand it back to her.

"Now, we can decide on your land. I got some listings in the areas you described as your dream location. Please, look over these and see if any of them are what you had in mind."

As you look through the real estate listings, you see so many perfect opportunities. They are exactly where you would want to build a dream home. You look at the surrounding areas and you can picture the beautiful landscape now. Hearing the local noises. Smelling the scents, feeling the peace it would bring to you to be there now. You realize you've held onto this particular listing for a while. You let her know this is the one you like the most. Her fingers fly across her phone as she informs you that the land now belongs to you. All the paperwork will be signed at the end. You are dumbfounded as you look at her and ask, "Why me? How did I know this man, why would he want to give me this dream life?"

"I don't know the details. I just know that your name was on his list, and it is the name that was selected. My job is planned out in exquisite details, which is why we are able to shuffle along through these tasks. You are in fact a very lucky person, with a great fortune. Let's not lose momentum now, the sooner we have everything in order, the sooner you get to experience your dream life. The best contractor and his team are prepared to draw up your dream house when you are ready. They will be here shortly, I have just sent them the land, so they will have a better idea on how to make things work for you. While we wait for them, are you happy in your current dwellings? Or do you want a new temporary home while your dream home is being constructed?"

You think long and hard on the question. Now that money is apparently not a problem, what do you want to do while your dream home is being constructed? Do you want to live here and just wait? Do you want to hire movers and move into a nice upscale place? Or a place far away from everyone and everything while you process your new life? Surely, you'll want to escape the media, if you stay in your current dwellings, you need people to help keep the media off you. Or maybe you'll step into the spotlight and shine, embracing your dream life. When you think of what you wanted you let the lady know and she assures you that nothing will be a problem. All your wishes for your new life will be answered.

The contractor has arrived with his team, only now that it is not just this lady in front of you, or the voice on the phone from earlier, the reality is really sinking in. Your life is going to become everything you've ever wanted. As they bring in their things and get settled you start to wonder what you will do with your life. With all your worries fading quicker and quicker into your past, what does your soul want? When everything material in this world becomes easily bought, what are the things you need to work on? How can you be the person that you truly want to be? Do you need all this money to accomplish your goals? Will it make your life that much easier? Probably, but when all those little inconveniences are covered, and no longer troublesome, does your life feel empty or is there a vast opening that you can now explore? Will you travel the world? Will you fund new charities or help those already established?

The contractor introduces himself and starts to ask questions about your dream home so that they may begin the process...you feel your mind flooded with images of beautiful houses, but you don't know where to start. You inhale and exhale and decide right now to start becoming the new you, as you describe this home. This home reflects who you are as a person. Build it from the ground up. Describe how you want your base, in detail, build your dream home, until you drift into a deep peaceful rest. When you wake up tomorrow, you will be this new person with a strong base to work on your dream life.

THE SECRET CABIN BEDTIME STORY

You have just left your car in the safe lot behind you. You walk upon the woods from the graveled lot, as you make your way onto the path you stop to admire the beauty. You close your eyes as you look up through the autumn leaves. Feeling the sunlight warms your face and smelling the crispness of the turned leaves. As the sunlight dances behind your eyelids you feel yourself calm and relax, ready to journey through this forest of warm sunshine and mellow color. Opening your eyes as you lower your head back you take in all the richness around you. Many of the trees are full with vibrant colors, some are evergreen, and some are showing their branches as their shaken off the old and are ready to embrace the new. You haven't explored this forest before, but you are going to meet a friend in a cozy cabin that is deep in the forest.

This small get away and escape from our technical world is exactly what you need. Taking a deep breath, you start to wander down the well-worn foot path. The path welcomes you as it has many strangers in the past. As you walk the leaves give a slight, satisfying crunch as your comfy hiking shoes cradle your feet. The once lush forest is in preparation for the upcoming winter. Just like your body settles in for the rest, it must prepare. As you feel your body settling into the autumnal shifts you notice the squirrels scurrying about, collecting their supply for their own long rest. The birds have mostly headed south and the only noise you can hear is the slight rustle of the leaves as a crisp wind blows through.

As you keep exploring into the woods, you come up on a large pine tree. You stop to admire it briefly, and you are amazed by the sheer size of it. This is the biggest tree you have ever seen. You cannot even see the very top, just lush and thick, deep green branches all the way to the top. You wonder how long this tree has been here. The things it must have been around to experience. Perhaps this tree was only a tiny sapling when your great, great ancestors were establishing the family that would eventually lead to you. Of all the cosmic events and paths of mother nature, one has led to you. Just like the many stages in your life they all have a beginning and an ending.

Nature is pleasantly predictable as all things follow a natural order, the sun rises, the sun sets, and a new day comes. You must rest in between to have a long, healthy life. This seed was planted. With nourishment it began to grow. Despite all odds, life continues. Saplings are able to grow into gigantic pine trees. You feel that slight breeze as it blows through and ruffles your hair, reminding you that you need to reach the cabin. You continue on the footpath... further from the city, closer to the still calmness of forest. The sounds of the city and busy roads are far behind you now. A distant memory as your body adjusts to the new sounds in the forest. Your body openly accepts the welcoming relaxation that the world is providing.

Your eyes relax with the warm colors surrounding you, the deep amber, the golden yellows, and the harvest orange of the leaves. You meander through the wooded land, and you notice a new sound. A pleasant sound of the faintest trickle of a babbling brook. As you travel closer to the brook you can see the stream flowing smoothly and calm, causing the smallest of waterfalls as the water caresses the round rocks. There is a striking green moss around the stream causing an ethereal appearance to this mystical place. The stream, clear and meandering, feels fresh, like it could wash away all your troubles just by being near it. Let the stream carry away any thoughts that are hindering you. Toss them into the stream and they can be washed away for another time. You watch your troubles slip away on the surface of the stream and you start to walk along beside the water.

As the stream wraps around the path, you see a small wooden bridge arcing over the pathway. Weather worn but sturdy, the bridge gives a little sigh as you walk across it. Holding on to the handrail you can feel the warmth from the sun radiating through your body. Though all this land is new for you, it oddly feels like coming home. Like the surrounding warmth you feel around you is familiar. It welcomes you with open arms and you wonder how much longer until you'll reach the cabin, how wonderful will it be? A little up ahead you can see a split in the path, as you get closer you can read the hand carved sign pointing to the right. Nightingale cabin is very close. Only a short distance to travel and you'll be ready for your vacation of peace and relaxation. The dense forest starts to give way to bigger rocks, hinting that you have explored yourself further to the edge of the mountain. To the left you can see as the vegetation has thinned out to make way for mountain cliffs, you will explore those later. For now, you just want to settle in.

Your pack starts to feel heavy on you. As if it has been weighing your body down with every step. Your legs long to rest, but you know there is not much further to go. Up ahead on the horizon you see the cabin. The green tin roof stands out against the autumn colors surrounding it. The welcoming warm woods and white trim make this cabin appear to be cozier than its grand scale depicts. The round logs only give way to grand white framed windows. Your tiredness turns into relief as you walk up the three short stairs to the welcoming door. Seeing a note on the door you read that your friend has gone out briefly but will return in a while. In the meantime, you are instructed to make yourself at home. You turn the knob and open the door, as you move through the threshold there is one sight that captivates you.

The large sightseeing windows provide a picturesque mountain overlook as you can now see the cabin is perched near a cliff. The colorful trees, spotted with occasional evergreens, is breath taking. You focus on your breathing as you look among the trees, breathing in, then slowly releasing that breath. How many different colors can you see? Breathing in you count 1, 2, and 3. Breathing out you count more. Do this until you've discovered all the colors there are to be seen in this beautiful forest that surrounds you. This welcoming home away from home.

You take off your pack and notice the kitchenette is to the left, the rooms off to the right, but directly ahead of you in front of the welcoming windows is a great room. You set your pack on the table by the entrance for now. You'll settle in with your things later. Now it is time to rest your body. The great room has a fireplace with wood and kindling ready to go, you notice the slight chill in the air so you decide starting a small fire is a good idea. You take the small logs from the top of the pile, along with some kindling, and place them into the fireplace. You notice the matches on a coffee table behind you and you use them to light this fire. As the small fire blossoms to life with a small roar and crackles you can feel the heat drifting off it. Feeling the warmth makes you realize there is a slight coldness that has seeped in from walking through the autumn forest. You look around the great room. Seeing the warm colors in the cabin reflecting those that are all around you in the woods.

There is an inviting brown leather sofa in the center of the room, with a deep red throw. You lie down on the sofa and sink down further into the comfort, pulling the throw around you and banishing all cold from your body. The warmth surrounding you as you hear the slight crackle of the fire. A light rain has started outside and you can hear the pitter patter on the green tin roof as you see the cold rain falling outside you are grateful to be inside. Warm and cozy, with softness snuggled all around you. As you close your eyes again you can feel the warm colors comforting your senses. The cabin is quiet, your mind is relaxed, and your body finally relaxes fully. Letting your arms down to your fingers drift off to sleep. Your neck and all down your spine, sinks into the sofa, relaxing on the most comfortable surface. Your legs all the way down to your toes sink further down off to sleep. Your mind drifts of to relax with the rest of your body. Let it relax, there is nothing holding you back. Your vacation starts now, your only job is to let everything slip away as your mind embraces the nothingness that is complete peace.

THE CUSTODIAN BEDTIME STORY

I was born in Oxford Aaron Jacobson on October 7th. 2018 in San Diego, California, to James Wilson Jacobson and Janine Anne Jacobson. Both of my parents were clairvoyant, as were both of their respective parents. I have "gifts" beyond those ever known in the modern history of the Earth. Some have called me a superhero because I help those in need and fight against oppression and hunger. Some have called me a savior because I speak in the xenoglossia and work with augury. I am, however, a mere mortal and desire no special treatment from any man.

When I was a newborn, I saw the trees swaying outside my nursery window and pointed to them when my parents were nearby. They understood and made a safe area for me to experience the natural surroundings of the outdoors. I loved the way the trees moved when the wind lightly fluttered through their branches. I marveled at the clouds and the non-linear formations and fractals that they endlessly created. I listened to the audible sounds of birds, insects, and other animals and understood what they were saying. I absolutely loved the colors of the planet that were everywhere in nature and the never-ending spiral curves of each component of it all. Non-geometric patterns, I noted, ruled growth and the manifestation of life.

When I was 4 years of age, my parents brought me a whiteboard and a chalkboard. They knew I would deliver arcane information. They wanted to know if I would choose the chalk or the dry erase pens. Both had placed their faith on the chalkboard, and that is the one I chose. On that chalkboard, I wrote the definitions of words that were never spoken. I set about the creation of machines to help the world operate on a cleaner and more efficient scale. I defined equations that led to the design and eventual manufacture of means of transportation and defense that revolutionized a great deal of what we see today, and I gave chemists, scientists, and surgeons, answers to how to prevent and illuminate physical conditions and detriments that, if left unanswered, would have caused mass pain and death in society's all around the globe.

When I was 10, the local police and detectives asked for my help with their work.

This I did to some degree but quickly learned that it was below my station and, after making accurate assessments of the problems and the nature of the issues they faced, I quickly located, trained and accredited other qualified individuals and instrumentally placed them in positions with the local and state police, as well as the FBI and in some cases, the government. After doing this, I placed myself into globally leaning endeavors in helping those in foreign lands who had been cut off from civil surroundings, and whose habitat had become severely compromised. Those were the victims of the power-hungry and the greedy who would use the backs of others to climb to temporary, pseudo heights. It is true that I do fight evil.

Today, I am the CEO of a multi-national corporation that creates software and equipment for large companies that build computing platforms and space systems. At least that is what the government believes. My venerate persona is crucially challenged by this deceit, and only the power of my mental armor protects me from the influence of guilt and shame in the name of honor among men of decree.

There are no insiders in my firm, only those who I hold dear, and their family members, understand what my intentions truly are. There are no visitors to the areas in my buildings which house the real workings of my business. It is a front. We do hire good normal people to create software, and we do make a profit from doing so, but all that is only a ruse to allow me to do what I do best. Help those who need help and those who cannot help themselves.

We make replicators and carry them to countries like Africa and farm equipment that produce accelerated growth crops inside of a week for those who have access to land but are repressed from otherwise doing so. Our labs are exclusive to this planet. We manufacture nanomachines that can build anything and do anything.

One top-secret area creates what we like to call peace machines. These are nanobots that slowly inhibit the bloodstream of those oligarchs who would serve only the health of themselves by trampling the rights and needs of others. They never know why they begin to get sick and slowly die, they just do, and then we go in and eliminate any remnants of their filthy existence so no history can ever know of their hatred and fears. These nanos are used with extreme care, and only when selected individuals are deemed impossible to rehabilitate. In that situation, only one platform is available. Regretfully, this is unanimous in its determination and its results.

My team personally travels with all the equipment in question and teaches the suffering masses how to operate these tools in a clandestine manner.

In this way, we are making strong communities in areas of the world generally dominated by greedy pea-brained thugs who love only power, money, and violence.

We also make a series of covert products that work by utilizing nanotechnology for medical purposes. Our technology has the power to easily re-grow limbs and internal organs, and regenerate beds that enable life extension. We apply these services, beginning at the bottom and moving up from there. The poor and homeless, the downtrodden and weak, always get what they need immediately. We are here to make lives better and push the evil global powers onto the ash heaps of history.

There is also one other piece of very valid and exclusive technology that we alone build that we do not sell or reveal to anyone else, and that falls into the area of time travel. When a tyrant shows up, and a timeline is initiated, we use our time tech to go back and prevent that tyrant from ever existing.

Now, I personally designed and assisted in the creation of something that could be called a weapon of peace. Before I explain what, it is and how we use it, I must tell you why we made it. Often times, in the work we do in various places around the globe, a person or group of people make plans or begin an agenda that, through some of our other technologies, we know will lead to the death or poisoning of a great many innocent people, sometimes a large portion of an entire culture in societies. The prime directive covering what we do and what I stand for does not and cannot allow these types of events to happen, so we neutralize them long before they can come to fruition. This brings us back to the way in which we do it.

It is called an Adapter Beam Machine. It looks like a very small chromium tube and can easily be an integral part of a soldier's gear. It can also be carried in one's pocket. It is that small! The beam unit is so incredibly powerful that only those with an extreme degree of psionics are even allowed to handle it, and those same individuals are exclusively qualified to carry and utilize it. The beam is activated with a sequence of mental acuity and memory and requires a system of codes.

When we are on a mission and intend to use the Adapter Beam, the codes are already inserted by the mission specialist who carries it, and it is ready to fire.

Generally, this unit is utilized in conjunction with time travel adjustment missions. First, we track the progress of something negative that happened. We determine the answer to the question, "What happened?" Then, we follow the timeline taking into consideration all the people whom that timeline touches, and we track it all the way back to its inception. In this way, instead of having to remove or neutralize an entire league of politicians, soldiers, or criminals, we only need to focus on one. Without the initial idea, the dominoes never fall!

In essence, what this amount to is prevention. Prevent the conception of the kernel of an idea from ever coming into manifestation, and you have prevented the negative results that the idea would have spawned.

In the end, here is how that looks. We learn that a certain devious and violent group is planning to overthrow a government that is working, which is a peaceful and productive institution. Then, we go back in time and use the Adapter Beam to discharge the individual who is responsible for the inception of that agenda, and we have removed the problem before it ever begins, thereby saving thousands, sometimes millions of lives. We think that is a good idea and a great service to the planet.

How is it that the Adapter Beam is the one technology that alone can do this? When the Adapter is discharged, there is a very powerful blue beam; call this a laser beam if you like, although technically, this would be incorrect. The beam enters the receiver's brain and de-develops the brain patterns giving them the mentality of a 10-year-old. They are not damaged or hurt in any way, but rather simply rendered ineffective. The carrier of the Adapter Beam weapon never goes into a mission alone, because after the shot, the receiver needs immediate attention. They become disoriented as the new brain patterns begin to send out sensory data, and, in some cases, the recipient may even need actual support, so they don't fall over and hurt themselves. My men are there in an instant! We bring this individual back with us and check them into special handling houses we have set up in various areas just for this purpose. In the course of a few months, they are placed back into society as janitors or night guards, something that requires little intelligence but provides a good degree of achievement on the part of the individual, while being totally innocuous in its essence. They are safe and well cared for during and after the entire ordeal. This is why the Adapter Beam Weapon is more a weapon of peace. The annihilation of a great many good law-abiding members of society is prevented, and a very bad person is rendered good, and can never ever have those negative thought patterns again for as long as they shall live. I am the custodian!

JOY BEDTIME STORY

Ruth was an elderly lady now, in her mid-seventies. She sat on her patio each morning, overlooking the neighborhood and waving to the people as they walked by. Each morning, children would walk to school and families would walk their dogs, and Ruth would just watch and smile at each one. This time of day was Ruth's favorite, as it reminded her of all of the wonderful things that she had to be joyful about in her lifetime.

Ruth remembered her childhood when she would walk to school with her six siblings and enjoy classes at the schoolhouse. She was not very fond of her teachers, but she loved learning, and she loved playing outside with her friends on breaks. She remembered sitting in the grass one afternoon eating a snack her Mom had packed for her and watching the younger kids play hopscotch in the dirt. To Ruth, this was one of her favorite memories that she shared with her siblings because it was so simple and brought so much joy to her life.

Ruth also remembered when she graduated and met her husband, Donald. Donald went straight into the military after school and served the country for nearly half a decade. For that entire time, Ruth raised their family, took care of the home front, and sent letters to Donald every week as she let him know how much she loved him and missed him. She would pour the day-to-day happenings into the letters, always trying to give Donald a feel of what was going on at home so that he felt like he was not missing out when he was gone. She remembered the sheer joy of seeing Donald for the first time, and for the first time after he returned home from every deployment. It always felt like she was falling in love all over again when he returned home.

Ruth also remembered what it felt like when Donald finally came home and stayed home, as he was done serving in the military. She remembered waking up to him every single day, learning how to live together as a couple, and living in sheer awe of this man who she adored so much. Ruth found so much joy in seeing Donald every day that she always did her best to find the small ways to bring even more joy into their days on a regular basis. Whether it was brewing him coffee when he was tired or slowly dancing with him in the kitchen, Ruth loved bringing a smile to Donald's face in any way that she could.

As an older couple walked by holding hands, Ruth remembered the joy she gained from holding hands with Donald all through his life. When they were walking in public, he would always grab her hand in his and lead her around, which helped Ruth feel so cared for and protected. She remembered how strong his hand felt, and how his body always seemed to be positioned in a way where he was ready to protect her if she needed him. Donald was a very protective and caring man, and Ruth always felt so safe in his presence.

Ruth remembered how even when Donald was ill with cancer, he was still so strong and protective until he could no longer be. As he withered away and he found that he was no longer able to protect Ruth physically, he still did his best to mentally and emotionally protect her by comforting her and telling her that everything would be okay. Donald told Ruth how he would watch over her every day so that she could carry on without him, even when she believed that she would never be able to. She was to wake up every day and continue looking for joy in every day, just as she had done since he had come home from the war. Donald told Ruth that she was to brew herself coffee, dance to their favorite songs while she sang quietly to herself and walk with bravery everywhere she went. This, Donald said, would be the way that she could feel his presence after he left.

Now, nearly twenty years after he had passed, Ruth still found ways to bring herself joy every morning. Part of that joy was in brewing herself a fresh pot of Donald's favorite coffee every morning and sipping a cup on the porch while she watched the families go by, while reminiscing on her own family that had long since grown and left. At night, she would put on their favorite songs and dance, or sing to them as she wiped off her makeup and prepared herself for bed.

As she was preparing to head inside for the day, Ruth saw an elderly couple walking their grandchildren to school. This made Ruth reminisce on her own grandchildren, and what it was like when they visited. When her children came to visit her, Ruth would share her favorite memories of Donald with them, in hopes of keeping his memory alive and introducing him to his grandkids through her memories. She would show them his photographs and watch them in sheer awe of how joyful they were to get to know the man that she had once loved so dearly, and in that she would find joy of her own. Every time, she knew that Donald was right there smiling with them and holding her hand, helping her stay brave whenever she missed him the most.

BRAZIL: RIO DE JANEIRO BEDTIME STORY

Before you begin your bedtime story, you will first need to center yourself and still and calm your mind. This part of the guided meditation will be very important to your nightly practice because without starting from a place of stillness, it will be difficult to let yourself completely engage with the story and get the maximum benefit from each carefully crafted guided meditation.

Take a long, deep breath in and exhale fully out. Breathe in again, this time pressing the tip of your tongue against the roof of your mouth, holding it there throughout the breath in. When you exhale, release the tip of your tongue and let it rest naturally in your mouth. Repeat this process, pressing the tip of your tongue against the roof of your mouth while you breathe in and releasing it on the exhale.

Continue this for at least one full minute, and then you will reverse the process. This time, you will breathe in a long, deep breath while letting your tongue relax and rest naturally in your mouth. Now, when you exhale, press the tip of your tongue against the roof of your mouth and hold it there throughout the entire exhale. Once you are ready to breathe back in again, let it rest naturally in your mouth. Continue this for at least one full minute.

The process of mind-body association is beneficial for teaching mindfulness and body awareness, which is an important aspect of anxiety and stress reduction. The benefit of reversing a physical association like this is that you are training yourself to be adaptable and amenable to different associations, which means that you are improving how quickly you are able to move in and out of anxious, panicky, and stress-filled states.

Everyone gets anxious or stressed on occasion. It is your ability to pull yourself out of this state that will make all the difference. Practices like this help to train you to be able to switch gears physically and mentally on command, and can be done anytime, anywhere, as often as you like.

Picture yourself on a busy street, filled and bustling with colorful costumes, lively music, and sprightly dancers. You are in Rio de Janeiro in Brazil, and you are at Carnival! There is a festive exuberance in the air as the dancers make their way down the street with lavishly decorated floats accompanying them.

The crowds that surround you are joyful and excited, and you would have to be made out of stone not to be affected by all of the excitement and revelry happening all around you! The Carnival of Rio de Janeiro is the largest carnival in the entire world, and the festival dates back to the 1700s. Some even refer to Carnival as the Biggest Show on Earth! Indeed, being here in the thick of it, it is easy to understand why it has earned that nickname. There are so many people here all around you, both participating in the actual parade and the spectators that are dancing, singing, and enjoying themselves from the sidelines.

The energy here in Brazil is absolutely electrifying, and you are reminded of the raw power of people getting together like this. There is something about a group of people joining together for a celebration that compounds excitement and happiness exponentially! It is a warm afternoon, and the sun is shining brightly down on all of the spectacularly decorated floats and the flamboyant and vividly colored costumes of the dancers.

The music keeps the beat, and you feel as if you are on fire, from your head to your toes and you are compelled to move along with the music. You look across at the people all around you. All ages, shapes, and ethnicities are out here to revel in the excitement of Carnival. There is a feeling of connection and community, and you are grateful to be here in the midst of this kind of celebration of life.

Life is meant to be embraced heartily and lived to the fullest. If you find yourself spending more time in survival mode than you'd like, remember that you can always find a celebration of life. You might find renewal and connection in a long lunch with a friend. You might rediscover the joys of being alive when you step out of your front door into the warm and welcoming sunshine of a fresh spring day. The world is full of life- affirming moments, but it is up to each person to take notice of them as they happen.

Let your mind drift back to your present reality. Take a long, deep breath while counting to three: 1 - 2 - 3 and back out 1 - 2 - 3. Again, deep breath in 1 - 2 - 3 and back out 1 -2 - 3. Do this as many times as you would like, letting your mind slowly come back to your present circumstances.

Remember, there is no invitation that will arrive for you to take notice of the many life-affirming moments that are taking place around you all day, every day. Your life is happening right now, and you have the privilege and the power to participate in any way you like. Can you think of a time that you felt rejuvenated and restored by participating in a celebration event or a personal connection of some sort? Your personal examples do not need to be grandiose or complicated- they just need to be yours. Let yourself remember the joyous celebration and connection you found in Rio de Janeiro, Brazil, and perhaps you may find yourself back there in your dreams...

Conclusion

We in general consider sleep when our mind and body shut down. Instead, sleep is a functioning period wherein a great deal of significant handling, reclamation, and reinforcing happens. Precisely how this occurs and why is still fairly a secret. In any case, we do know the importance of benefits of sleep, and the reasons we need it for ideal well-being and prosperity. Hypnosis is tricking your body in order to produce something good about your body, we can use it in our daily lives, or even in our sleeping patterns.

I have used inspiration from many self-hypnosis sessions I have followed online to improve my own mindfulness. There's a special level of satisfaction you gain from the time and effort you invest in yourself. You will feel proud of yourself for taking the long and narrow road. Remember that hypnosis works overtime, you'll grow stronger with every session you complete. Some sessions are useful to repeat a few times, reminding yourself of your newly gained information.

Think about the information you have gained in this audio guide. You have learned to open yourself to new people and new adventures. You can never know if you will enjoy something until you've tried it. The night you decided to stay home instead of going to the club could have been the night you would have met your life partner. You could even have met your best friend. Do you really want to live with regret? You only have one life, make the most of it.

I think of my pilot friend who I mentioned in the fifth session. I look up to him today. It's been a few years now, but he is a huge inspiration to me. He recognized an addiction as something that makes him happy for five minutes at a time and replaced it with a hobby that has shown him the world. I love listening to his stories when I see him. He always has some interesting adventure to talk about in a place I haven't even heard of. I'm just going to admit it; I envy him a little.

I explained the techniques I combined in the overall introduction, but I know some of these sessions seemed harsh and others might have frightened you for a moment. My objective was simply to help you visualize a problem before defeating it by using the three combined methods. I don't support the idea of regression hypnosis. I believe in focusing on where you want to be and not where you used to be. I have seen the effectiveness of this approach myself. It gives new meaning to scaring the issue out of someone.

I once had a patient who was terrified of clowns. I used a similar approach with him as my test run when I started hypnosis. I could feel the sweat dripping from my chin as I thought he was going into shock. He wasn't relaxed at all; he wasn't mindful enough to face his fear. I can remember jumping up to open the curtains and let fresh air into the room. I had never seen a patient as bleak as I saw him that day. I admit that it took some time to regain his trust. He would reluctantly come in for sessions and refuse any hypnosis. I made it my goal to study hypnosis and perfect my unique technique of making the person's fear visualization before helping them conquer it. I'm proud to say that he gave me one more chance to try my new technique. I understood hypnotic state better and proceeded confidently. I brought him to his ultimate calm before making him face the clown. Long story short, he can take his children to the carnival without having an anxiety attack now.

We wish you success in your endeavor to seek peaceful sleep.

Printed in Great Britain
by Amazon